Contraception

To our children
and grandchildren

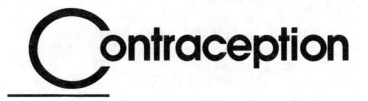

Contraception

A Guide to
Birth Control
Methods

Vern L. Bullough, R.N., Ph.D., and **Bonnie Bullough,** R.N., Ph.D.

Prometheus Books Buffalo, New York

Product photographs appear where indicated courtesy of the manufacturer or supplier. The authors emphasize that these photographs are for informational purposes only and in no way constitute an endorsement of the brand names shown. Original drawings by Steven Bullough.

Published 1990 by Prometheus Books Publishers
700 East Amherst Street, Buffalo, New York 14215

Library of Congress Cataloging-in-Pulication Data

Bullough, Vern L.
    Contraception : a guide to birth control methods / Vern L. Bullough, Bonnie Bullough.
        p.   cm.—(New concepts in human sexuality)
    Includes bibliographical references.
    ISBN 0-87975-589-X
    1. Contraception—Popular works. I. Bullough, Bonnie.
II. Title. III. Series.
RG136.2B85   1990   65573   RG   89-49202
613.9′4—dc20   136.2
                                                B85   CIP
                                                1990

Printed on acid-free paper in the United States of America

Contents

5

Preface

The purpose of this book is not only to give information about various forms of family planning but to help the reader understand the long struggle that led to today's availability of various forms of birth control. We believe that the ability of women to plan their pregnancies · has been one of the most dramatic developments in human history. While we strongly believe that such planning is best when both parties are involved, it is the woman as childbearer for whom it was proclaimed that "biology is destiny." It is the ability to plan pregnancies, or entirely avoid them, that has so challenged the traditional concepts of the role and status of women in society, and has helped to make the relationship between the sexes more equal. Women will continue to bear children, but we hope that ever-increasing numbers of them will be wanted children and not simply accidental by-products of sexual intercourse.

Steven L. Mitchell, our editor, came up with the idea for this book and guided it through the various stages of publication. Bruce Carle and his able staff did the typesetting. The cover design and placement of illustrations are the work of Valerie Ferenti-Cognetto. Many of the illustrations were drawn by Steven Bullough especially for this book. Special thanks are also due to those publishers and pharmaceutical companies who have given their permission to reprint and/or supplied photographs and illustrations appearing in this volume.

1

Information You Always Wanted to Know

Under favorable circumstances it is estimated that the average woman could become pregnant every other year during her reproductive life, which is roughly between 15 and 45 years of age. This would mean that the average woman, provided she did not give birth to twins or have other forms of multiple births, would give birth to fifteen children during her lifetime. However, some women would become pregnant more often, others less often, with a theoretical maximum of about twenty pregnancies for one woman. But what is theoretical is not always actual. The largest number of live births recorded for any one woman is sixty-nine by the first wife of Feodor Vassilyev (her name does not appear in the records), a peasant from the village of Shula, 150 miles east of Moscow. She had twenty-seven pregnancies; but included in these were sixteen pairs of twins, seven sets of triplets, and four sets of quadruplets born between 1725 and 1765. Almost all of these offspring survived beyond their first year.[1]

The most prolific mother of the twentieth century is Leontina Espinosa Albina (b. 1925) of San Antonio, Chile, who by 1988 had produced 59 children, including five sets of triplets. Forty of her children, 24 boys and 16 girls, were alive at that time. Though most pregnancies result in only one infant, it is possible to have more. Records show that several women have given birth to 10 infants in one delivery, most of them stillborn before term. Several have given birth to nine (nontuplets), some of which have survived. The highest number of births where all survived is the case of sextuplets, three males and three females, born to Mrs. Susan Jane Scoones Rosenkowitz on

October 28, 1947, at Mowbray, Cape Town, South Africa. Similarly, while few women beyond their middle forties bear children, some have become pregnant at later ages. There are several undocumented cases of women in their seventies having children. Historians have been reluctant to accept such cases because in those which have been most closely investigated, it turns out the mother or grandmother was claiming as her own an illegitimate child of a daughter, granddaughter, or even great-granddaughter. The oldest mother for whom satisfactory verification is available gave birth (to a daughter) at the age of 57 years and 129 days. This was Mrs. Ruth Alice Taylor Shephard Kistler (1899–1982) whose daughter Suzan was born in Glendale, California, on October 18, 1956.[2] It is also possible to get pregnant at a fairly young age, although this is unusual. Several pregnancies have been recorded for girls under the age of ten.

If a male had children every time he engaged in sexual activity, he could impregnate thousands of women and have thousands of children. Though this in fact does not happen, at least one man in history had over a thousand children. The male who is recorded to have fathered the most children is the polygamous Moulay Ismail (1672–1727), the last Sharfan Emperor of Morocco. He was reported to have 525 sons and 342 daughters by 1703, and in 1721 he recorded the birth of his seven hundredth son. Apparently he no longer counted the number of his daughters.[3] The Western male with the most progeny was probably Augustus the Strong (1670–1733), King of Poland and Elector of Saxony. His nickname came from his ability in the bedchamber and not from his military skills; he was the father of 365 children, only one of whom was legitimate, his successor, Augustus III (1696–1763). Among the most famous of his illegitimate children was Maurice de Saxe, who became a marshal of France.[4]

Theoretically, when a couple engages in intercourse without using contraceptives or methods to calculate when ovulation occurs (and the woman is not already pregnant), there is a three percent chance that pregnancy will occur. In simple terms, this means that, on the average, pregnancy results once every thirty-three or thirty-four times the couple engages in intercourse.

Though we have little data for men on their past frequency of intercourse, Alfred E. Kinsey and his associates found that the period of greatest sexual activity in married American males occurs between the ages of sixteen and twenty. The younger married males engaged in intercourse more than 3.0 times a week, compared to 1.7 times a week for the age group forty-one to forty-five.[5] By implication, the age of the male partner has some bearing on how many pregnancies a woman will have since not only is intercourse less frequent with older men but the sperm count also declines as men age. Similarly, the older the woman at marriage, the fewer pregnancies she will have since she is fertile for fewer years. One form of birth control then is having men and women marry at considerably older ages, as is the custom in Ireland, although this also assumes that the woman will not engage in any sexual activity until she is ready to marry. Such assumptions are not usually made about the sexual activity of men, who are free to visit prostitutes or engage in temporary liaisons. The delay in marriage works most effectively in countries with strong double standards of sexual conduct or where government or religious control and interference in the private lives of its citizens is the greatest.[6] Similarly, polygamy also tends to cut down the number of children each woman has simply because of the inability of one man, at least in those places where it exists on a large scale, to realize the full potential of so many wives.[7] Even though the record for most children is held by the polygamous Moulay Ismail, his harem included hundreds if not thousands of women.

Few, if any, individuals or societies have ever approached the maximum level of fertility, and the conclusion seems obvious that various customs and methods have been adopted to limit the number of births. Statisticians like to talk of a "total maternity ratio," which could be defined as the average number of previous live births per woman now aged forty-five or over, regardless of whether a particular woman has children (not all women can or do have children). This ratio varies with different groups and societies. For the Ashanti of Africa the total maternity ratio has been estimated at approximately six, for the Sioux Indians eight, and for certain groups of Eskimos less than five. Only a minority of people have ever approached a rate as high as ten.[8] The highest rate recorded in history is 10.6 among the Hutterites in the first half of the twentieth century. The Hutterites are a communal religious group dating from the sixteenth century who settled in South Dakota between 1874 and 1877. They now live in over a hundred different religious colonies in the Dakotas, Montana, and Washington in the United States, and Alberta, Saskatchewan, and Manitoba in Canada.[9]

Note that the "total maternity ratio" is based upon live births, which means that abortions are excluded whether they are spontaneous or induced. Being born alive, however, does not mean that the infant survives to reach adulthood. Though infant mortality figures of the past are notoriously difficult to determine accurately, it is estimated that somewhere between 25 and 40 percent of the infants born alive prior to the nineteenth century did not live beyond their first birthday.[10]

Though infant mortality certainly cuts down population growth, it is not a form of birth control. Still, there is considerable evidence that the high mortality rate of newborns in many societies has not always been due to natural causes but has resulted from actions that would either consciously or unconsciously have led to a high death rate. Though few individuals and societies deliberately murder their infants (infanticide), various policies subtly (and some not so subtly) encourage it. A good example of this is the practice of wet nursing as it existed in the eighteenth and nineteenth centuries in Paris and elsewhere. Infants who had survived the first three or four weeks (during which mortality is the highest) were removed from the mother and sent to the country to be fed by other women who usually kept them for a year or more. Since wet nurses by definition usually had infants of their own to feed, and the parents of the boarded infant did not live close, the care varied tremendously and the mortality rate was very high, much higher than it would have been had the birth mother fed her own infant. One study estimated that of those infants sent out to wet nurses, some 25 percent had died by the end of the year. This would lead to a total mortality rate of over 40 percent.[11]

Perhaps the most obvious way to avoid either becoming pregnant or getting someone pregnant is to remain celibate. This in essence was the Christian remedy, and lifelong celibacy is still encouraged among such groups as Catholic priests and nuns. In the past, however, only a few societies have been either willing or able to impose long periods of celibacy upon more than a small minority of their members. Instead, most societies in the past were content to adopt short periods of continence by imposing prohibitions upon sexual intercourse during certain times of the year such as Lent, various feast days, or during certain periods of a woman's life (e.g., when she is lactating or menstruating). It is highly unlikely that such prohibitions originally were established as birth control measures, although they undoubtedly helped to cut down the pregnancy rate. The modern rhythm method is a deliberate effort to utilize periods of temporary continence to cut down the possibility of conception, but its effectiveness depends not only on understanding the menstrual cycle, something that we have only recently begun to do, but on the ability of any particular woman to determine when she ovulates, something that was impossible in the past and is still not easy (more will be said on this later).

Throughout history, people have also tried to utilize artificial means of preventing conception, although only a few have been particularly effective. Contemporary peoples who still live in tribal or nomadic groups, for example, are known to use douches and drugs, to practice withdrawal (*coitus interruptus*), and to insert tampons and pessaries, all to avoid pregnancy. Sub-incision is also practiced in some groups, and has a long history, although whether it was originally done for ritualistic reasons or contraceptive purposes is not now clear. Sub-incision is an operation that creates a hole in the male urethra at the base of the penis near the scrotum so that during ejaculation semen dribbles over the scrotum instead of entering the vagina. A more normal ejaculation can be obtained by covering the hole with a finger which acts as a plug and allows the semen to follow its original path. When he urinates, the male also must put his finger over this hole, otherwise the urine will come from it and dribble all over him.[12]

The oldest known contraceptive prescriptions date from the second millennium (between 2,000 and 1,000) B.C.E.* and come from Egypt. These call for the use of such substances as crocodile dung, honey, and gumlike substances, some of which would have been partially effective if inserted into the vagina and if a woman could bring herself to use them. Others, however, would have been less effective. Modern research, for example, has found that those women who overcame their inhibitions about crocodile dung suppositories and used them would not have found them very effective in preventing pregnancy since the alkaline dung would have neutralized the acidity of the vagina, thus creating optimum conditions for sperm. These suppositories, however, might have proven effective in discouraging the male partner from wanting intercourse in the first place. Still other recipes calling for such ingredients as elephant dung would

---

*Before the Christian Era

have been much more effective as contraceptives because their composition is more acidic than crocodile dung. These statements are based on modern laboratory studies that perhaps are somewhat misleading since the alkalinity or acidity of any of the various suppositories would have been modified by the materials with which they were mixed, and to our knowledge none have been tested through clinical trials.

Honey or oily substances have long been recognized for their contraceptive properties and have been widely used throughout history. The ancient Greeks, for example, utilized olive oil. All similar oily substances tend to act as an impediment to the movement of sperm, although such methods were never infallible. Some of the traditionally used substances, however, were more effective than others. For example, one of the gums often used in ancient prescriptions was gathered from the tips of the acacia shrub and contained considerable lactic acid, an ingredient ultimately used in many contraceptive jellies.[13]

Various intrauterine devices (IUDs) also have a long history of use by women to prevent pregnancy. Books attributed to Hippocrates, the founder of Western medicine, mention their existence in ancient Greece; and on a more practical level, Arab camel drivers were accustomed to inserting a round stone into the uterus of a female camel before departing on a long journey in order to prevent her from becoming pregnant. Occasional references to IUDs also periodically crop up serendipitously in the medical literature. This is because a physician would report finding objects in the uterus or vagina of a woman who had come to him for treatment of a gynecological problem. (Usually, in the past, gynecological matters were left to the expertise of the midwife, and only the most persistent problems were seen by a physician.)[14]

One of the more effective ancient contraceptives was the insertion of a sponge soaked in vinegar or wine before engaging in coitus. This method is mentioned in the Talmud some five times and once more in the Tosefta, and might have been used by the ancient Egyptians as well. The term used in the Talmud is *mokh,* and the commentators indicate that it could be used by (1) a minor who otherwise might become pregnant and die; (2) a pregnant woman since, it was believed, the penetration of semen into the uterus might cause a spontaneous abortion; and (3) a nursing woman who might otherwise become pregnant and have to wean her child prematurely.[15]

With the exception of sub-incision, the methods so far rely upon the female rather than the male to adopt some means of preventing conception. This generally seems to have been the case throughout much of history, although there are references to methods that the male can use. One obvious method that some couples today still practice is *coitus interruptus*, where the male withdraws before achieving orgasm. Though some semen escapes from the Cowper's glands before the male ejaculates, and thus pregnancy is always a theoretical possibility even with the most devoted followers of this method, it is condemned by Jewish, Christian, and Islamic commentators for other reasons. This is because in much of Western thought it traditionally has been regarded as a sin for a male to waste his seed. The belief is based upon the following statement in the Book of Leviticus:

> And if any man's seed of copulation go out from him, then he shall wash all his flesh in water, and be unclean until the evening. And every garment, and every skin, whereon is the seed of copulation, shall be washed with water, and be unclean until the evening.[16]

Obviously this passage can refer to a spontaneous emission (a "wet dream"), premature ejaculation, and masturbation, as well as *coitus interruptus*. The prohibition is spelled out in more detail in Genesis and the story of Onan:

> And Judah said unto Onan, Go in unto thy brother's wife, and marry her, and raise up the seed to thy brother. And Onan knew that the seed should not be his, and it came to pass, when he went unto his brother's wife, that he spilled *it* on the ground, lest that he should give seed to his brother. And the thing which he did displeased the Lord: wherefore he slew him also.[17]

Though Talmudic and other commentators debated the meaning of this, they felt in general that it did not prevent the use of contraceptives on the condition that the sexual pleasure of the woman was the object. They, however, were more inclined to look favorably on contraceptive barriers used by the woman. Islam was also tolerant of contraception, preferring to interpret the statement as a violation of Allah's command rather than a generalized sexual act. Christians of various varieties, however, have utilized the story of Onan and the other biblical references to condemn not only the use of contraceptives but any sexual act not leading to procreation.[18] In spite of opposition to *coitus interruptus,* there was a strong tradition within Catholic theology tolerating *coitus reservatus* in which intercourse takes place but without ejaculation. This is not a sure fire method of preventing pregnancy, however, since some semen can dribble out without ejaculation.

The first so-called modern contraceptive device to be described was in fact designed for the male. This is the sheath or condom, first described by Gabriele Fallopius in the sixteenth century. Fallopius (1523–1562) also was the first in medical literature to describe the clitoris as well as the tubes that bear his name. In addition, Fallopius is well known for his studies on venereal disease, and it was in this connection that he described the male sheath:

> As often as man has intercourse, he should (if possible) wash the genitals, or wipe them with a cloth; afterwards he should use a small linen cloth made to the glans, and draw forward the prepuce over the glans; if he can do so, it is well to moisten it with saliva or with a lotion; however, it does not matter; if you fear lest caries [syphilis] be produced [in the midst of] the canal, take the sheath of this linen cloth and place it in the canal; I tried the experiment on eleven hundred men, and I call immortal God to witness that not one of them was infected.[19]

Whether Fallopius invented the condom or was describing an experiment on a method long used before is debatable. The sheath, in fact, might be one of those items that are invented a number of different times for a variety of purposes and their contraceptive value was only incidental to these other reasons. One of the earliest stories of the possible use of such a device appears in the Greek legend of Pasiphaë and Minos. Minos had a serious problem in that his initial ejaculate contained serpents and scorpions that either injured his partner or prevented conception. To solve his problem he was advised to slip a goat bladder in the vagina of a woman. Using this he cast off this serpent-bearing semen before turning to Pasiphaë, whom he successfully impregnated.[20] Probably the original inventor of the condom must remain unknown, although Fallopius certainly helped popularize it. In 1597, a certain Hercules Saxonia suggested improving Fallopius' linen sheath by soaking it several times in a chemical solution, then allowing it to dry in the shade. Other suggested improvements included the use of animal intestines as well as fish bladders as materials for making the sheath. The condom was initially intended primarily as a prophylactic device designed to cut down the possibility of contracting venereal disease rather than as a means of preventing conception, although its contraceptive properties were also recognized.

In England, the sheath came to be known as a condom for reasons that have eluded scholars, although all sorts of mythological explanations have been advanced. Most center around a mythical Dr. Condom, allegedly a physician at the court of Charles II (1660–1685) who supposedly invented it, but no such person has ever been found in the records. Like most things dealing with sexuality, the condom had a variety of euphemistic names. The English often called it the "French letter," while the French called it *la capote anglaise* or "the English riding coat." Whatever the name, condoms were widely used in the better houses of prostitution during the eighteenth century.[21] The famed womanizer and diarist Giovanni Jacopo Casanova de Seingal (1725–1798) used them extensively, both as prophylactics and as contraceptives. He tested them beforehand by filling them with air. James Boswell (1740–1795, the famed biographer of Samuel Johnson) also mentions them. Condoms were constructed of various materials during the eighteenth century, but those made from part of the large intestine of lambs, sheep, calves, goats, and perhaps other animals were particularly favored. The difficulty with condoms was in part economic, since they were fairly expensive until the mass-produced rubber ones appeared in the nineteenth century. This meant that they were often used over and over and, unless they were washed carefully, could become disease carriers.

Details on various prophylactics will appear in later chapters of this book, but it was not until the twentieth century that effective contraceptives really developed. The problem was to find an effective means that was neither too expensive nor too inhibiting to the aesthetics of the sex act. Once such a method was found, it was also necessary to disseminate the information. One of the major obstacles to the development of effective contraceptives was the lack of scientific knowledge about reproduction. Though it is obvious that during orgasm the man secretes a serous whitish fluid, and the correlation of this fluid with pregnancy has been recognized throughout recorded history, it was not until the development of the microscope that it was realized that semen contained sperm. For many centuries Western ideas about conception were essentially those promulgated by

Aristotle in the fourth century B.C.E., who held that even though both sexes were important in the reproductive process, man was the more active partner since he contributed the semen, while the woman only contributed the material for the semen to work upon.[22] Building upon Aristotle, the Arabic medical writer Avicenna compared the whole process of gestation to the making of cheese, with the male sperm equivalent to the clotting agent in milk, while the female "sperm" was compared to the coagulum. Still, the key starting point remained the male semen.[23] In Western Europe, St. Albertus Magnus (in the thirteenth century) went so far as to argue that females came about from a weaker seed than males: if the seed material was well digested and strong, the creation of males would result, but if it was poorly digested and weak, it resulted in "femalization" (and the birth of a girl).[24] Such an attitude reinforced beliefs about the inferiority of women because it was believed that they derived from weaker seeds.

Better understanding of the process was dependent upon more effective knowledge of the human body. In this the anatomical work of Andreas Vesalius in the sixteenth century proved important, as did Gabriele Fallopius's more specialized studies on female anatomy. Fallopius outlined not only aspects of the female reproductive system never before described, but also the male *arteria profunda* which dilates and brings blood to support the erection of the penis. Even with these more detailed anatomical studies, there was a widespread belief that the uterus itself was more or less independent of the woman, almost an animal within her, floating free in her body cavity, and on occasion causing hysteria and other such "female" diseases.

This belief about the supremacy of the male in procreation was finally challenged by William Harvey (1578–1657), whose *Anatomical Exercitations Concerning the Generation of Living Creatures* was published in Latin in 1651 and in an English translation in 1653. Harvey had observed the hatching of hens' eggs and had carried out experimental anatomical studies on the deer in the royal deer park. From his studies he arrived at the conclusion that the one reproductive principle common to all living creatures was the ovum or egg. This view was summarized later by the Swedish biologist Carl Linnaeus (1707–1778) as *vivium omne ex ovo*—literally, "everything living comes from the egg." Other biologists came forth with supporting conclusions, particularly Marcello Malpighi (1628–1694), whose study of the embryo in hens' eggs was published in 1672. At about the same time, Reynier de Graaf (1641–1673) observed the changes taking place in rabbits' ovaries in the first days after fertilization and concluded that similar changes probably took place in the human female.

The growing influence of the "ovists" ran into a roadblock in the studies of Anthony van Leeuwenhoek (1632–1723), whose observations, made possible through the newly invented microscope, were not equaled until the nineteenth century. Johan Ham, a medical student, brought Leeuwenhoek a glass bottle containing the semen of a man who suffered from nocturnal emissions. Ham had observed "animalcula" or little animals in the semen and he wanted Leeuwenhoek to confirm his findings. Leeuwenhoek not only did so but reported that these little creatures were different from other animalcula he had seen. He said they were distinguishable by their round bodies with tails five or six times as long as their bodies and that they made swimming movements like an eel. He then put them aside to look at them again, but when he attempted to do so a few hours later he found they were no longer moving, although they were still clearly recognizable. To make certain that these little animals were not the result of any sickness, Leeuwenhoek, along with Ham, proceeded to examine the semen of healthy males and found the same kind of creatures. Leeuwenhoek estimated that there must be a thousand or more confined within the space of a grain of sand. As their observations continued, it was found that the animalcula died within twenty-four hours if kept in cold temperatures, but if they were kept in warm conditions, they survived several days. It was Leeuwenhoek who called these animalcula *spermatozoa,* the name by which they are now known. The results of his discoveries were published in the *Proceedings of the British Royal Society* in 1678 and almost immediately examining semen became a popular pastime. One observer reported that in examining the semen of a horse, he had actually seen miniature horses, while another reported that the semen of the donkey was filled with miniature donkeys. Still others thought they could distinguish female sperm from male sperm, and some went so far as to say they saw male and female sperm copulating, then giving birth to little sperm. The effect, in spite of some of the ludicrous tales, was to reassert, in the minds of many, the supremacy of the male. Part of the difficulty was that although the ovary was easily observable, the mammalian ovum was very difficult to observe. It was not until the nineteenth century that Karl Ernst von Baer (1792–1876) found the egg cell in a mammal. Finally in 1877, a Swiss biologist, H. Fol, observed the entry of the sperm into the ovum of the starfish, thus making it possible to understand the whole process of fertilization in rough outline.[25]

With such misconceptions about the nature of fertilization, it was natural that contraception was often endowed with magical connotations. It was widely repeated in European folklore that if a woman threw objects such as kernels of grain, apples, stones, wooden pegs, or nails into a well, spring, or river, she would remain free from pregnancy. Another superstitious belief held that if a woman turned the wheel of a grain mill backward four times at midnight, pregnancy would be averted; while still another popular folk belief held that if a woman walked over the graves of her dead sisters calling out three times "I don't want any more children," pregnancy would be avoided.[26]

Though it came to be assumed during the later part of the nineteenth century that the female carried an egg which, when fertilized, led to her becoming pregnant, there were still misconceptions about how this happened. It was believed that menstruation had something to do with it, but how and in what ways was unclear. Though we have a vision of the dispassionate scientist continually establishing new frontiers of knowledge, not all scientific writing is done by dispassionate scientists or even based upon research. Much of it in the past, and some of it today, is not so much science as what might be called advocacy, and in the nineteenth century the push for greater freedom for women coincided with new breakthroughs in the understanding of human physiology. Sometimes, however, breakthroughs were announced which in the light of today's knowledge seem simply to have been reactionary opinions cloaked in the mantle of science. For example, a physician named A. F. A. King published an article in the journal *Obstetrics* in 1875 claiming that menstruation was pathological—in effect, an illness. He held that in the biblical paradise known as the Garden of Eden, humans had reproduced asexually. It was only through eating the fruit of evil, and man's subsequent fall from grace, that perfection had been replaced by the evil of sex. King believed that intercourse during the menses was dangerous, forbidden, and resulted in gonorrhea. Yet he also believed that it was at this very time that conception was most likely to occur. Since menstruation therefore stood in the way of fruitful coitus, it obviously was contrary to nature and not ordained by God, since no god would have made woman contagious at the same time she was most fruitful.[27]

King's concept was radically different from the view put forth in earlier popular sexual manuals such as the pseudonymous *Aristotle's Masterpiece,* which explained that menstruation was the casting out of excess blood that would have nourished the embryo had pregnancy occurred.[28] In his own way, King was trying to apply modern scientific discoveries to challenge old (and in this case more accurate) information, but he was doing this in a very unscientific and moralistic manner. He based his condemnations on the findings of a German, E. F. W. Pflüger (1829–1910), who in 1861 had demonstrated that a woman whose ovaries had been removed did not menstruate. In trying to explain this finding, Pflüger had hypothesized that the growth of a follicle in the ovary at a certain stage in its development produced a mechanical stimulus of the nerves that triggered menstrual bleeding and ovulation. From this Pflüger came to believe that menstruation and ovulation occurred simultaneously.[29] It was not until the twentieth century that the involvement of hormones in the timing of ovulation was fully understood. In the meantime, many physicians accepted Pflüger's theory that nervous stimulation triggered menstruation.

This erroneous belief in the existence of a "nervous" trigger of menstruation led a number of physicians and pseudoscientists to express opposition to any emancipation for women since the physiological necessity of developing the nervous system of females, so essential for reproduction, made it next to impossible for their bodies to also develop intellectual powers (also believed to be part of the nervous system) at the same level as men. This was because men could concentrate all their energy on developing their intellectual powers. In short, biology was destiny, and inevitably such assumptions led to a belief in the natural intellectual inferiority of women and their inability ever to compete successfully with men in the intellectual world.[30]

Another factor to be considered in any discussion of contraceptives is the difficulty that early research pioneers experienced when attempting to disseminate information. This is still a problem, since any discussion of contraception must of necessity involve a discussion of sex, a topic not yet considered fully respectable by large segments of the population. In fact, the struggle to disseminate information about the existence and availability of the contraceptives mentioned in this and later chapters was not particularly successful until well into the twentieth century. The history of these efforts at public awareness is a checkered one and the ultimate success is due to two more or less conflicting groups who became interested in the problem: (1) the radicals who saw the continuous burden of childbirth as destructive to women and who realized that large families in an industrial society were a cause of poverty rather than a support as they had been in earlier agricultural societies, and (2) the eugenicists, most of whom were upper-class people who believed that the world's resources were limited and that unless the poor "stopped breeding" and the rich increased their reproductive rate, civilization would collapse. Though this is a somewhat oversimplified view, it does help to explain how the movement to popularize contraception developed as well as some of the current debate.

Both groups looked to the Reverend Thomas Robert Malthus (1766–1834) and his anonymous *Essay on the Principle of Population,* originally published in 1798. Malthus, who believed that human beings were possessed by a sexual urge that led them to multiply faster than their food supply, finally signed his name to the second and expanded edition published in 1803. According to Malthus, the inevitable result of this unchecked sexual urge was misery, war, and vice—unless some checks were applied. This was because population would increase geometrically (1, 2, 4, 8, 16, 32 . . .) while food supplies would only increase at an arithmetic rate (1, 2, 3, 4, 5, 6 . . .). His solution: humans must bridle their sexual instinct. Malthus himself was opposed to any mechanical restraints to intercourse; instead he urged humans to restrain their sexual instincts and marry as late as possible. Sexually, Malthus was an extreme conservative who went so far as to classify as vice all promiscuous intercourse, "unnatural" passions, violations of the marriage bed, use of various contraceptive devices, and irregular sexual liaisons.[31] It was because Malthus opposed the use of contraceptives that those who supported his belief in the need for population control but deviated from his prescribed plan by advocating the use of contraceptives came to be known as Neo-Malthusians.

Much of the early information about contraception was passed from mother to daughter or, if printed, put out in the form of throwaway tracts designed to reach the widest possible audience. The contraceptive movement in the English-speaking world is generally dated from the proposals of the English tailor Francis Place (1771–1854), who was concerned about the widespread poverty he saw. To help overcome this state of affairs through limiting the number of children, Place published his *Illustrations and Proofs of the Principle of Population* in 1822. He urged married couples to use "precautionary means" in order to better plan their families, but he did not go into detail. To remedy this lack of instruction, in 1823 he printed handbills addressed simply *To the Married of Both Sexes,* describing a way to avoid pregnancy. He advocated the insertion of a "piece of sponge about an inch square" into the vagina "previous to coition." This sponge was to have a double twisted thread or bobbin attached to it so it could later be withdrawn. Users were advised to dampen and warm the sponge before insertion.[32]

Place's pamphlets and those of a similar nature by some of his contemporary disciples were never subject to any legal interference, although they were brought to the attention of the attorney general. After a time, Place turned to other issues and the initial effort to disseminate effective birth control information was dropped. The next phase of the movement emerged in the United States in 1831 with the publication by Robert Dale Owen of a booklet titled *Moral Physiology.* Among other things, Owen discussed three methods of birth control: *coitus interruptus,* the vaginal sponge, and the *baudruche* or condom. He favored *coitus interruptus* because, in his mind, the vaginal sponge was not always successful and the condom (then made of animal intestines) was much too expensive and unpleasant to use. He reported that a good condom cost about "a dollar" and could only be used once. He did, however, recognize the effectiveness of the condom in' preventing sexually transmitted diseases.[33]

More controversial was Massachusetts physician Charles Knowlton's booklet *Fruits of Philosophy,* originally published in 1832. Though it was ultimately very influential, initially Knowlton's birth control methods were not equal to his influence. Knowlton was a great advocate of douching, which consisted of

> syringing the vagina, soon after the male emission into it, with some liquid, which will not merely dislodge nearly all the semen, as simple water would do—the female being in the most proper position for

the operation—but which will destroy the fecundating property of any portion of semen that may remain.[34]

To achieve this end, Knowlton recommended a douching solution of alum with infusions of almost any available astringent vegetable substance such as white oak or hemlock bark, green tea, or raspberry leaves, although alum alone would do if nothing else was available. In some cases, he recommended the use of sulfate of zinc in combination with alum salts. Actually alum as a spermicide would have been a fairly effective contraceptive, although zinc sulfate would not. Even for alum to be effective, however, it would have to be used almost immediately following intercourse, and it is doubtful that Knowlton's advise was very effective. His advocacy of both a potentially effective spermicide douche and a not very effective one indicates the basic lack of knowledge possessed by people of the time.

Knowlton, however, is not so much remembered for his contraceptive advice, inadequate as it was, as for the difficulties he faced in disseminating it. In 1832, he was fined at Taunton, Massachusetts, and in 1833 he was jailed three months in Cambridge for distributing the book. A third attempt to convict him in Greenfield, Massachusetts, led to disagreement among two different juries and the case was dropped. Needless to say, attempts to censor Knowlton's work only served to publicize it, so that by 1839 it had sold over 10,000 copies. Other editions, both legal and pirated ones, appeared throughout much of the century mostly through a kind of underground distribution system. This was true of other works on contraception that appeared during the rest of the century. The most notable exception was George Drysdale's *Elements of Social Science,* originally published in England in 1854, a comprehensive treatise on sex education with only 5½ pages of the 449-page book devoted to contraceptives. Still, his was the most comprehensive discussion of the subject at that time. Drysdale included five different techniques: he advised that the preferred method was the sponge inserted before intercourse, followed by a douche with tepid water. He also recognized a so-called sterile period, placing it from two to three days before menstruation until eight days after, but he did not suggest that intercourse was totally without risk of pregnancy on these days. Drysdale felt that *coitus interruptus* was physically injurious, interfered with pleasure, and caused nervous disorders. He dismissed the sheath or condom as unesthetic or resulting in reduced enjoyment and/or potential impotence.[35]

Giving a new impetus to the birth control movement in the last part of the nineteenth century was the growth of the eugenics movement. Though this grew out of the Malthusian concern over excessive population growth, the eugenicists voiced concern primarily about the high birthrates among the poor and the illiterate, and the low birthrates among the more intellectual upper classes. Eugenics, in fact, defined itself as an applied biological science concerned with increasing the proportion of persons of better-than-average endowment in succeeding generations. The word had been coined by Francis Galton (1822–1911), a great believer in heredity. Unfortunately, he also had many of the prejudices of an upper-class Englishman in regard to social class and race. Galton's hypotheses were given further "academic" respectability by Karl Pearson (1857–1936), the first holder of the chair of eugenics, which had been endowed by Galton at the University of London. Pearson believed that the high birthrate of the poor was a threat to civilization, and if members of the "higher" races did not make it their duty to reproduce, they would be supplanted in time by the members of the "lower" races. When put in this way, eugenics gave "scientific" support to those who believed in racial and class superiority. It was just such ideas that Hitler attempted to implement in his solution to the "racial" problem. Although Pearson's view was eventually opposed by the English Eugenics Society, the American Eugenics movement, founded in 1905, adopted his views. Since the eugenicists also believed in the widespread dissemination of information about contraceptives, a segment of the organized planned parenthood movement often included eugenicists. The beliefs of the Pearson-oriented eugenicists and their presence in various groups advocating contraception has sometimes led to the denunciation of Planned Parenthood as an elitist organization trying to cut down the growth of minority and poor populations. For example, during the 1970s, one group of black militants condemned all contraception as racial genocide.

Even without the burden of the early eugenicists' belief in racial and class superiority, the birth control movement often found it difficult to contact the people it most wanted to reach, namely the poor, overburdened mothers who did not want any more children. This was because, following the passage of the first laws against pornography in 1853 in England, information on contraception was interpreted to be pornographic since, of necessity, it included a discussion of sexuality. In 1868, Sir Alexander Cockburn issued the so-called Hicklin decision, a judicial opinion holding that the test of obscenity was whether "the tendency of the matter as obscenity is to deprave and corrupt those whose minds are open to such immoral influences and into whose hands a publication of this sort may fall."[36] Books containing contraceptive information—works such as Knowlton's that had been sold for decades in England—were seized and the booksellers convicted of selling obscene literature.

The guilty verdicts led to a concerted attempt by free thinkers to challenge English obscenity law by reprinting the Knowlton book and publicly announcing that they would sell it. Two of those involved, Charles Bradlaugh and Annie Besant, were brought to trial. Sir Alexander Cockburn, who was again the trial judge, held that though there had never been a more ill-advised or injudicious prosecution, he nonetheless was bound to explain the law to the jury. The jury returned a rather unusual verdict in that they found the book to be "calculated to corrupt public morals" but exonerated the "defendants from any corrupt motives in publishing it." Cockburn held that this was a guilty verdict, which caused some consternation to members of the jury who thought they were voting for acquittal. Bradlaugh and Besant were sentenced to serve from two to six months in prison and pay a fine of 200 pounds. On appeal the conviction was quashed on the grounds that the indictment itself was erroneous. The net result of all this was a growing public awareness of the existence of the possibility of contraceptives; and with Bradlaugh and Besant's acquittal on a technicality, books and pamphlets on contraception became widely available in England and there were no further prosecutions.

Americans were not so fortunate during the post-Civil War period, which saw a growing movement to provide "moral guidance" for the vast numbers of young people flocking to the expanding urban centers. The result was the formation of societies such as the New York Society for the Suppression of Vice, the Boston Watch and Ward Society, and similar groups in other major urban centers. One of the issues of great concern to such societies was the growth of "pornographic" literature, and one of the first successes of the new groups was the 1873 tightening of postal laws regulating obscenity. Anthony Comstock, the secretary of the New York Society, managed to get himself appointed a special postal agent, and for the next forty years he acted as a moral censor for material disseminated through the mails.[37]

One of the first works to run afoul of Comstock was a pamphlet titled *Words in Pearl for the Married,* so called because it was printed in pearl type. Its author was Edward Bliss Foote, a strong advocate of contraception. Included in the pamphlet was a discussion of methods of birth control, and it was this that led to Foote's prosecution in 1876 and to his subsequent conviction in the U.S. District Court of New York. He was fined $3,000, more than most people earned in a five-year period. Though no known copy of his pamphlet has yet turned up in a major research library, from other sources it is known that Foote advocated the traditional condom made from animal intestines or fish bladders (which he held were much better) and also a new type of condom made from India rubber—it was fitted just over the end of the penis and was called an Apex Envelope. In addition, Foote advocated a "womb veil," also made of India rubber, which was designed to fit over the cervix. Furthermore, he supported douching. Foote peddled something called an "Electro-Magnetic Preventative Machine," which would allow men and women to engage in intercourse without fear of pregnancy, but it is hard to reconstruct the machine's specific nature.[38]

With Foote's successful prosecution, contraceptive information went underground in the United States. Inevitably, few Americans, except those who went to Europe regularly, kept up with contemporary developments such as the diaphragm, which began to be prescribed in Dutch clinics at the end of the nineteenth century. The few physicians who did keep current in the field tended to restrict their services to upper-class groups. The change in this situation is generally credited to a nurse, Margaret Sanger (1883–1966).

A militant socialist, Sanger in 1914 began to publish a magazine called *The Woman Rebel,* the aim of which was to stimulate working women to think for themselves. Toward this end, she announced in the magazine that she would defy the laws pertaining to the dissemination of contraceptive information. In 1914, she proceeded to publish a small pamphlet, *Family Limitation,* for which she was arrested. Though she attended the preliminary hearing, Sanger fled to Europe before her formal trial. During her absence (much of which she spent learning about European contraceptive methods), her husband, William Sanger, who had little to do with his wife's publishing activities, was arrested and convicted after being tricked into giving a copy of the pamphlet to a Comstock agent, a young women who pleaded with him for information on how to avoid pregnancy.

The arrest and conviction mobilized a group of women, the best known of whom was Mary Ware Dennett. These women organized the National Birth Control League in 1915, demanding a change in laws regulating the flow of information about birth control. In the meantime, Margaret Sanger, upset at her innocent husband's conviction, returned to America, determined to stand trial and give further publicity to the existence of birth control. The government, however, after several delays, refused to prosecute. Undoubtedly one of the reasons for the declining interest of the government in prosecution was the death of Anthony Comstock, to whose activities increasing numbers of people had been opposed. Emphasizing this opposition was the large number of prominent people from all over the United States who had come to Margaret Sanger's defense.

Sanger was relieved at being free from prosecution but still anxious to spread the message of birth control. To reach the working women, Sanger; her sister Ethel Byrne, also a nurse; and two social workers, Fania Mindell and Elizabeth Stuyvesant, opened a birth control clinic in Brooklyn in 1916, one patterned after the Dutch clinics. The well-publicized opening attracted long lines of interested women as well as several vice officers. After some ten days of disseminating information and devices, three of the women—Margaret, her sister Ethel, and Fania Mindell—were arrested. Mrs. Byrne was tried first and sentenced to thirty days in jail. She promptly went on a hunger strike that attracted national attention and after eleven days she was pardoned by the governor of New York. Fania Mindell was also convicted but was fined only $50. By this time the courts were willing to drop charges against Margaret Sanger provided she would agree not to open another clinic. She refused and was sentenced to thirty days in jail, but immediately appealed her conviction. The Court of Appeals gave a rather ambiguous decision, holding that it was legal to disseminate contraceptive information for the "cure and prevention of disease" but failed to specify the disease. Sanger, interpreting pregnancy as a disease, continued her campaign through this legal loophole and was not challenged.[39]

New York, however, was just one state, and there were numerous other state laws to be overcome. Even when the legal barriers began to fall, public policies of many agencies made it difficult to distribute information. Volunteer birth control clinics were also prevented from publicly advertising their existence. In fact, it was not until 1965 that the U.S. Supreme Court, in the case of *Griswold* v. *Connecticut,* removed the last obstacle to the dissemination of contraceptive information. Since then it has been legal to distribute such information in all fifty states. The problem, however, still remains one of disseminating accurate information, and that is the purpose of this book.

NOTES

· 1. *Guinness Book of Records, 1989,* edited by Donald McFarlan (New York: Sterling Publishing, 1988).

2. Ibid.

3. Ibid.

4. John B. Wolf, *The Emergence of the Great Powers* (New York: Harper, 1951), p. 76.

5. Alfred E. Kinsey, Wardell B. Pomeroy, and Clyde E. Matin, *Sexual Behavior in the Human Male* (Philadelphia: W. B. Saunders, 1948), pp. 336, 356, tables 81 and 88.

6. "Age at Marriage and Fertility," *Population Reports* Series M. Number 4 (November 1979), Vol. 7, No. 6.

7. For the effect of polygamy see H. V. Muhsam, "Fertility of Polygamous Marriages," *Population Studies* 10 (1956–1957): 3–16.

8. Clive Wood and Beryl Suitters, *The Fight for Acceptance* (Aylesbury, England: Medical and Technical Publishing Company, 1970), p. 10.

9. Even the Hutterite ratio, however, has declined in recent decades. See J. W. Eaton and A. J. Mayer, "The Social Biology of Very High Fertility among the Hutterites: The Demography of a Unique Population," *Human Biology* 25 (1953): 206–64; L. M. Laing, "Declining Fertility in a Religious Isolate: The Hutterite Population of Alberta, Canada, 1951–1971," *Human Biology* 52 (1980): 289–310; K. A. Peter, "The Decline of Hutterite Population Growth," *Canadian Ethnic Studies* 12 (1980): 97–110.

10. Richard Harrison Shyrock, *The Development of Modern Medicine,* 2d ed. revised (New York: Alfred A. Knopf, 1947), p. 102.

11. See George D. Sussman, "Parisian Infants and Norman Wet Nurses in the Early Nineteenth Century: A Statistical Study," *Journal of Interdisciplinary History* 7 (Spring 1977): 637–53; Sussman, "The Wet-Nursing Business in Nineteenth-Century France," *French Historical Studies* 9 (1975): 304–28.

12. Norman E. Himes, *Medical History of Contraception* (reprinted, New York: Schocken Books, 1970), pp. 41–51.

13. Ibid., 59–80.

14. Woods and Suitters, *The Fight for Acceptance,* p. 107

15. For a more complete discussion see David M. Feldman, *Birth Control in Jewish Law* (New York: New York University Press, 1968), pp. 174–75. For citations see *Yebamot,* 12b, 100b; *Ketubbot,* 39a; *Nedarim,* 35b; *Niddah,* 45a, and *Tosephta Niddah,* i, 6.

16. Leviticus 15:16–18. All biblical references are from the Authorized Version (King James' Edition).

17. Genesis 38: 8–10.

18. For a discussion of this see John T. Noonan, Jr., *Contraception: A History of Its Treatment by the Catholic Theologians and Canonists* (Cambridge, Mass.: Belknap Press of Harvard University Press, 1966).

19. This is a translation by Himes's *Medical History of Contraception,* pp. 176–77.

20. The story appears in Antoninus Liberalis, *Metamorphoses* 41, in *Mythographi Graeci* (Leipzig: Teubner, 1894–1902).

21. See Vern L. Bullough and Bonnie Bullough, *Women and Prostitution* (Buffalo, N.Y.: Prometheus Books, 1987).

22. Aristotle, *Generation of Animals,* 728A, 17 ff.; 1729A, 25–34; 766 A., 1935, trans. A. L. Peck (London: William Heinemann, 1953).

23. Avicenna, *Canon of Medicine,* I, 196, trans. O. Cameron Gruner (London: Luzac and Company, 1930), p. 230.

24. Albertus Magnus, *De Animalibus Libri XXVI,* edited by Hermann Studler (2 vols., Munster: *Beitrage zur Geschichte des Mittelalters,* vols. 15 and 16, 1916–1920), lib. IX, tract 2, cap. 3, pp. 714 ff.; lib. XV, tract 2, caps. 4–11, pp. 1026 ff. See also Claudius Franz Mayer, "Die Personallehre in der Naturalphilosophie von Albertus Magnus," *Kyklos,* II (1929): 191–257, and Paul Dipegen, *Frau and Frauenheilkunde in der Kultur des Mittelalters* (Stuttgart: George Thieme Verlag, 1963), pp. 149–51.

25. See Joseph Needham, *A History of Embryology* (New York: Abelard Schuman, 1959), and Clifford Dobell, *Anthony van Leeuwenhoek and His "Little Animals"* (New York: Russell & Russell, 1958). See also F. J. Cole, *Early Theories of Sexual Generation* (Oxford, England: Clarendon Press, 1930).

26. Himes, *Medical History of Contraception,* pp. 176–77.

27. A. F. A. King, "A New Basis for Uterine Pathology," *American Journal of Obstetrics* 8 (1875–1876): 242–43.

28. Aristotle (pseud.), *The Works of Aristotle in Four Parts, Containing I. His Complete Master-piece; . . . II. His Experienced Midwife; . . . III. His Book of Problems; . . . IV. His Last Legacy . . .* (London: Published for the bookseller, 1808), p. 126. For a discussion of this see Vern L. Bullough.

"An Early American Sex Manual," *Early American Literature* 7 (1973): 236–46.

29. E. F. W. Pflüger, *Über die Eierstöcke der Säugethiere und des Menschen* (Leipzig: Engelmann, 1863).

30. Vern L. Bullough and Martha Voght, "Women, Menstruation, and Nineteenth-Century Medicine," *Bulletin of the History of Medicine* 47 (1973): 66–82.

31. Thomas Robert Malthus, *An Essay on the Principle of Population,* 2d ed. (London, 1803), p. 11.

32. For a discussion of Francis Place and a biographical sketch see Peter Fryer, *The Birth Controllers* (London: Secker and Warburg, 1965), pp. 43–57, 72–74; a reproduction of a surviving handbill is published in Himes, *Medical History of Contraception,* pp. 216–17.

33. Fryer, *The Birth Controllers,* pp. 92–93, and Himes, *Medical History of Contraception,* pp. 224–25. The booklet had sold approximately 60,000 copies by 1874.

34. Charles Knowlton, *Fruits of Philosophy,* edited by Norman E. Himes and Robert Latou Dickinson (Mount Vernon, N.Y.: Peter Pauper Press, 1937), p. 60.

35. Himes, *Medical History of Contraception,* pp. 233–34, and Fryer, *Birth Controllers,* pp. 110–11.

36. Norman St. John-Stevas, *Obscenity and the Law* (London: Secker and Warburg, 1956), pp. 70, 126–27.

37. See Paul S. Boyer, *Purity in Print* (New York: Charles Scribner's Sons, 1968).

38. The description comes from Foote's book *Medical Common Sense Applied to the Causes, Prevention and Cure of Chronic Diseases and Unhappiness in Marriage* (revised and enlarged edition, New York: Published by the Author, 1866), pp. 378–81. In later editions of the book this section was removed and apparently published separately, and it was this, or a version of it, that was seized by Comstock.

39. There are many biographies of Margaret Sanger, including an autobiography written in 1938 and republished in 1971. See *Margaret Sanger: An Autobiography* (reprinted, New York: Dover Books 1971).

2

Some Anatomy and Physiology
You Should Know

Pregnancy occurs when an egg is fertilized and then implanted into the lining of the uterus. Traditional methods of contraception were for the most part what are called barrier methods since they attempted to erect a barrier between the egg and the sperm, thereby preventing the two from coming together. Other methods were devised to eliminate sexual intercourse when the egg is in the fallopian tubes ready for fertilization. Later, more scientifically sophisticated methods were aimed at preventing the implantation of an egg by one means or another. Approaches such as sterilization eliminate either the sperm or the egg depending on which sex is sterilized. Ultimately, if these various attempts to prevent pregnancy failed, then abortion (whether in the past or today) has been the last resort for dealing with unwanted pregnancies.

MALE ANATOMY AND PHYSIOLOGY

In simple terms, the male reproductive system consists of a pair of testes that produce sperm and hormones, a network of ducts designed to transport the sperm from the testes to other points on their journey, a variety of glands that produce semen, and the penis. The testes are egg-shaped structures located in the scrotum, a sac-like structure that hangs outside the male body at the base of the penis. Physio-

31

logically the testes are located in the scrotum because it is cooler than the abdominal cavity, where a higher body temperature would (as in undescended testicles) destroy the sperm. The average testicle measures one to one and half inches in length, and each manufactures and secretes the hormone testosterone as well as small amounts of estrogen, the female hormone, and androsterone, another male hormone. Within the scrotum each testis (or testicle) is suspended at the end of what is called the spermatic cord. The cord contains blood vessels, nerves, a sperm duct called the *vas deferens,* and a thin muscle called the *cremaster* muscle, which encircles each testicle and raises it closer to the body in response to fear, cold, anger, and sexual arousal. Each testicle contains hundreds of structures called *seminferous tubules* where sperm is produced. If these tightly coiled tubules were stretched out, they would extend one to three feet in length. At the back portion of each testis is the *epididymis,* a storage and excretory unit for sperm. Its smooth walls contract when ejaculation takes place, moving the sperm out into the connecting tube or vas deferens. The vasa deferentia (both of which are severed when a male is sterilized) run along the testicle, up into the abdominal cavity, and around the bladder before emptying into the *ejaculatory ducts,* which enter the prostate gland. It is here that sperm from each testicle is combined with fluid from the prostate gland to produce the semen that enters the urethra. The urethra in the male serves double duty, functioning as a carrier not only of the semen but also of urine.

The sexual process that starts with arousal causes the penis to change from its flaccid resting state to an erect condition called tumescence. This is possible because the penis includes two cylinders, *corpora cavernosa,* made up of spongy tissue. Cells in this tissue have spaces between them and arousal causes the space to fill with blood. With further stimulation of the tumescent penis from intercourse or other sexual activity ejaculation occurs and semen is expelled from the urethra.

The ejaculate of the average male contains from 200 to 400 million sperm, but the sperm only account for about one percent of the total volume of the semen. In addition to fluid from the epididymis, the seminal vesicles, and the prostate gland, semen also contains secretions from the Cowper's glands. These glands flank the urethra and empty into it through tiny ducts. It is believed that the alkaline

MALE REPRODUCTIVE SYSTEM

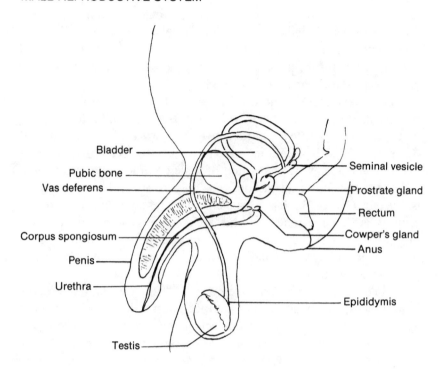

Bladder
Pubic bone
Vas deferens
Corpus spongiosum
Penis
Urethra
Testis

Seminal vesicle
Prostrate gland
Rectum
Cowper's gland
Anus
Epididymis

CROSS-SECTION OF A MALE TESTIS

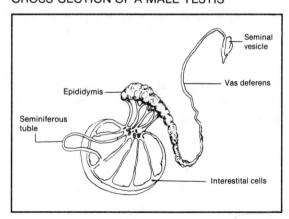

Seminal vesicle
Vas deferens
Epididymis
Seminiferous tuble
Interestital cells

Illustration by Steven Bullough

secretion of the glands helps neutralize the acidity of the urine in the urethra, thus making possible the survival and mobility of the sperm. Cowper's glands also contain a small number of sperm (proportionately smaller though the number is still in the millions), and this pre-ejaculatory fluid can impregnate a woman even if the man withdraws before ejaculation takes place.

Obviously there is more to the anatomy and physiology of the male than this brief overview, but these essentials indicate the ways in which male-oriented contraceptives can work. The male barrier contraceptive is the condom, which prevents the semen from entering the vagina. The other method of male contraception widely used today is sterilization: the vas deferens going from each of the testicles is severed. One of the basic problems with research on male contraceptives is that the male is fertile all the time and not periodically or cyclically as is the case with the female, and so the problem is to find ways to control male fertility during those periods when pregnancy is not desired.

Male fertility, however, does decline with age. This is because in healthy males the secretion of androgen begins declining from about age thirty until age sixty, after which it remains relatively constant. The decline in androgen secretion brings about several physiological changes. The seminferous tubules, the site of sperm production, begin to thicken and deteriorate slightly. Sperm production itself begins to decline at about age fifty-five, although normal sperm is still produced. As the androgen secretion declines, the size and firmness of the testicles diminish, and they do not elevate to the same degree for sexual activity. The seminal fluid becomes thinner and ejaculatory pressure decreases. The prostate gland often enlarges and its contractions weaken. Consequently, the pregnancy rate resulting from unprotected intercourse declines but it is still possible for men of advanced age to father children. Senator Strom Thurmond, the conservative Republican senator from South Carolina, for example, fathered his fourth child at age seventy-four. As the male ages, more time is needed to achieve an erection, which is sustained for shorter amounts of time following ejaculation. The interval between orgasm and subsequent erection and ejaculation also lengthens, and after age sixty some twelve to twenty-four hours might elapse before penile erection once again can be attained. Ejaculation is also likely to involve seepage rather than the explosive contractions of the younger male.[1]

FEMALE ANATOMY AND PHYSIOLOGY

The female reproductive system is not as visible as that of the male. It consists of a pair of ovaries, two fallopian tubes, a uterus, cervix, vagina, and vulva. The ovaries are almond-shaped organs located in the pelvic cavity, nestled in the curve of the fallopian tubes. Ovaries are the female counterpart of testes and in fact develop from similar tissue during the fetal differentiation between male and female, a process that takes place within a few months of conception. Both ovaries and testes produce reproductive cells (eggs and sperm respectively) and both secrete hormones. The ovaries primarily produce estrogen and progesterone although they also secrete small amounts of masculinizing hormones including testosterone. At birth the ovaries contain between 230,000 and 400,000 ovarian follicles, clusters of nutrient- and hormone-secreting cells with an immature egg in the center. Only 400 to 500 of these eggs, or ova, will be released from their follicles, one each month, from puberty until menopause.

Each fallopian tube, which is connected to the uterus, is about four inches long. The end of the fallopian tube nearest the ovary is not connected to it directly. Instead it has a funnel-like opening with fingerlike edges (called *fimbria*) that help the ovum enter the tube through a process not yet fully understood. Inside the tube are hairlike structures known as *cilia* that sway in the direction of the uterus and guide the ovum along. The tube also contracts to help push it along. Fertilization, if it takes place, occurs in the fallopian tubes near the entrance closest to the ovaries.

The uterus resembles an upside-down pear and is held suspended in the pelvic cavity by a series of ligaments. It is located between the bladder and the rectum. It shifts and contracts in response to pregnancy, the filling or emptying of the bladder or rectum, and during sexual intercourse. The walls are partially composed of smooth muscles; it is the contraction of these muscles that occur during orgasm, childbirth, and during menstruation. The contractions during menstruation are more pronounced (and painful) in some women than in others.

At the lower end of the uterus is the cervix, which extends into the vagina. It has an opening or mouth (referred to as the *os*) through which sperm can enter the uterus and travel up to the fallopian tubes. It is also the opening through which childbirth takes place.

FEMALE EXTERNAL GENITALS

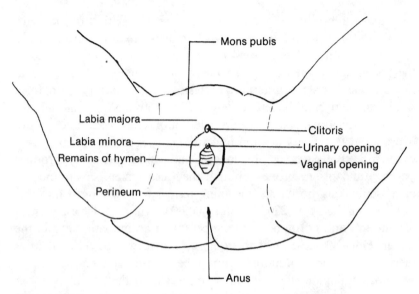

Mons pubis

Labia majora
Labia minora
Remains of hymen

Clitoris
Urinary opening
Vaginal opening

Perineum

Anus

FEMALE REPRODUCTIVE SYSTEM

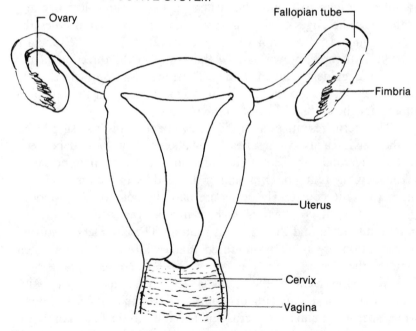

Ovary

Fallopian tube

Fimbria

Uterus

Cervix

Vagina

Illustration by Steven Bullough

The cervix has glands that excrete varying amounts of mucus. This mucus plugs the entrance to the cervix and forms a barrier against the entry of sperm during most of the menstrual cycle. During ovulation the mucus is thinner and more permeable.

The vagina is a thin-walled muscular tube that extends from the uterus to the external opening, which is called the *introitus.* The walls contain many blood vessels that become engorged with blood during sexual excitement and during childbirth. Under congestion or pressure from the blood, small amounts of fluid are squeezed through the cell walls. This fluid acts as a lubricant during sexual intercourse and delivery. The process is very similar to that which leads to arousal in the male.

The *vulva* is the term usually given to the external genitalia of the female including the *mons pubis,* the outer and inner lips (*labia*), the *clitoris,* the *introitus* or vaginal opening, and the urinary opening (entrance to the urethra). The mons pubis is a cushion of fatty tissue covering the pubic bone. It is covered with pubic hair and has a large number of touch receptors. The *labia majora* (outer lips) cover the external genitalia; they merge with the rest of the body skin at the back at the *perineum,* the area between the anus and the labia. In the front they come together a small distance above the clitoris. The labia majora are similar to the scrotum in the male and have fewer touch and pressure receptors than the mons. The *labia minora* (inner lips) are the inner covering for the vagina. They are thinner than the outer labia and have no hair on them. They enclose both the vaginal and urethral openings as well as the ducts of the Bartholin glands, which produce a small amount of mucus. The clitoris, anatomically similar to the prepuce or foreskin of the penis, is one of the most erotically sensitive parts of the female body. It is permeated with both pressure and sensory receptors.

The female reproductive system includes two physiological processes, menstruation and childbirth, which are exclusive to the female. All other physiological processes are shared in common between the sexes. Unlike male fertility, which is relatively constant during the productive years, female fertility is cyclical and involved with the menstrual cycle. Ovulation occurs normally about once a month and is regulated by pituitary hormones. Menstruation itself is regulated by ovarian hormones, namely, estrogen and progesterone. Estrogen is the major hormone active in female development, and it is the finely tuned regular intervals of estrogen and progesterone secretion that control the menstrual cycle.

Menstruation usually takes place about every twenty-eight days but most women have variations of this with both shorter and longer cycles. Every month during the reproductive years one of the ovarian follicles (or occasionally more than one) matures. Triggering this growth to maturity are secretions of estrogen from one of the cell layers in the follicle. These have been activated by the hypothalamus, which signals the pituitary gland to secret the follicle stimulating hormone (FSH) and this stimulates the primordial follicle to begin developing. The follicle with the maturing egg moves toward the surface of one of the ovaries (usually ovulation alternates between each ovary), whereupon the ovarian surface disintegrates, allowing the egg to float out into the abdominal cavity where it is picked up through the funnel-shaped end of one of the fallopian tubes and begins a journey of about six and a half days to the uterus. Occasionally a few drops of blood or follicular fluid may fall into the abdominal cavity. This irritation produces a cramp on either the left or right side of the lower abdomen or lower back, depending on which side the ovary is located. This cramp, sometimes very painful, is known as *mittelschmerz,* which means "middle pain." On rare occasions the pain is also accompanied by a bloody discharge in the vagina. Usually during both the day before the egg is discharged and the day after, the cervix excretes a clear, stretchy mucus.

Just before ovulation the same cell layer in the follicle starts secreting progesterone as well as estrogen. These hormones are secreted by the *corpus luteum,* the term used for the follicle after ovulation. Literally, the term means "yellow body," so named because of the yellow fat in it. These hormones help maintain the pregnancy if it has occurred. The estrogen secreted by the corpus luteum causes the uterine lining (*endometrium*) to proliferate. This involves a growth of new cells and glands that secrete nourishing substances for an embryo. At the same time, the progesterone secreted by the corpus luteum increases the uterine blood supply and causes these small glands so recently formed in the endometrium to begin secreting nourishing substances. The lining expands until ovulation takes place and progesterone is secreted whereupon the lining becomes secretory. A fertilized egg can only be implanted in a mucus-rich secretory lining, not a proliferating one. If fertilization does not take place, the amount of both estrogen and progesterone produced by the corpus luteum declines, and after about twelve days ceases altogether. When this happens the arteries and the veins in the uterus slow down their flow to this new lining, and most of it, what is known as the superficial endometrium, is dislodged and expelled. It is this shedding process that causes menstruation since it is evacuated from the uterus and through the cervix into the vagina. Once menstruation is complete, the whole process starts over.

The menstrual cycle is the key to many of the new methods of contraception, and both the birth control pill and the IUD utilize it in different ways to prevent pregnancy. Natural family planning methods also rely upon the cycle to calculate when a woman will not be fertile. The barrier methods available to women—such as the diaphragm, cervical cap, and the sponge—are designed to prevent entry of the sperm into the cervical canal.

As in the male, female physiological processes are also affected by aging. In women estrogen production begins to decline at about age forty and continues until about age sixty. Menstruation itself ceases in most women between forty-five and fifty-five years of age. Other physiological changes also take place. The steroid-deprived walls of the vagina become thinner, the acidic secretions diminish, and the rate of production of vaginal lubrication also lessens. Even before the estrogen production begins to decline, there are processes that take place which make it more difficult for women in their mid-thirties to carry a pregnancy successfully to term or which increase the probability of having a genetically abnormal child (such as one with Down's Syndrome). This is why amniocentesis is performed much more often on women who are pregnant and past the age of thirty-five. Theoretically it is still possible for a woman to become pregnant right up to the time she finally ceases ovulation, so to avoid conception some form of contraception remains important.[3,4]

NOTES

1. For a discussion of these changes see W. H. Masters and V. E. Johnson, *Human Sexual Responses* (Boston: Little Brown and Company, 1966), pp. 259 ff.

2. J. Smolev, "Male Reproductive Anatomy and Physiology," in

Men's Reproductive Health, edited by J. M. Swanson and K. A. Forrest (New York: Springer Publishing Co., 1984), pp. 31–46.

3. A. R. Allgeier and E. R. Allgeier, *Sexual Interactions,* 2d ed. (Lexington, Mass.: D. C. Heath and Company, 1988), pp. 93–115.

4. Boston Women's Health Book Collective, *Our Bodies, Ourselves: A Book By and For Women* (New York: Simon and Schuster, 1979), pp. 24–37.

3

Barrier Contraceptives

Barrier methods of contraception rely on placing some kind of obstacle in the vagina to prevent the passage of sperm into the uterus. It is both a modern and a traditional method of pregnancy prevention. Some of the historical attempts to establish a barrier employed materials similar in shape to those currently used.

In Sumatra, for example, women molded opium into a cuplike shape and inserted it into the vagina to cover the cervix. Chinese and Japanese women covered the cervix with oiled silky paper (*misugami*), while Hungarian women used beeswax melted into 5 to 10 cm. disks.[1] Some historical barrier devices were quite ingenious. Giovanni Casanova, whose *Memoirs* record his numerous sexual conquests, recommended that women squeeze half a lemon and then insert the lemon rind into their vaginas, fitting it over the cervix. In today's terms the lemon rind would act as an obstructive cup while the citric acid remaining in the pulp would serve as a spermicide.[2] This principle is the basis for those barrier methods used today that are under the control of the woman. The problem is to make sure that the cup stays in place (that would not always have been the case with the lemon rind); and present-day spermicides are far more effective than the lemon juice.

Rubber, even before techniques had been developed to vulcanize it, was widely used in the form of *pessaries*—devices inserted into the vagina to support a prolapsed (fallen) uterus or for alleviating symptoms of abnormal retroversion (a backward displacement of the uterus), anteversion (anterior displacement of the uterus), anteflex-

41

PESSARIES

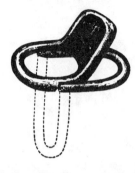

Thomas's anteversion and anteflexion pessary

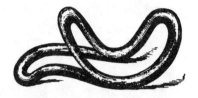

Thomas's elastic pessary for anterior displacements

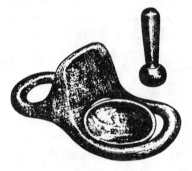

Anteflexion pessary supporting intra-uterine stem

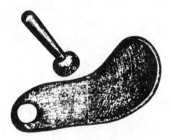

Glass stem supported by disc pessary

Thomas's anteversion pessary as it appears in the vagina

The same instrument as it appears on removal

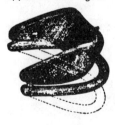

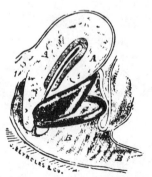

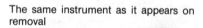

The same instrument in position

PESSARIES (CONT.)

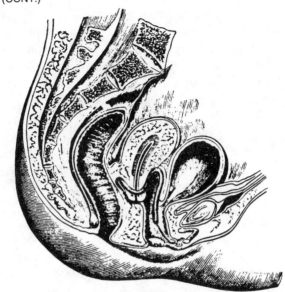

Graily Hewitt's anteversion pessary

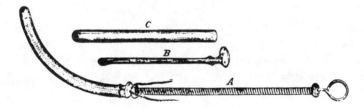

Campbell's soft-rubber spring-stem pessary. A. The soft-rubber stem and spring prepared for introduction. B. Shows the spring separately. C. The rubber cap or hood.

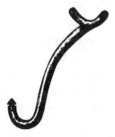

Cutter's T pessary for anterior displacements

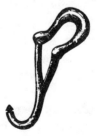

Thomas's modification of Cutter's pessary

ion (bending forward of the neck of the uterus), or similar problems. Since a tipped uterus does not ordinarily cause problems, the variety of devices designed to deal with such conditions is puzzling to today's readers. If, however, they are seen as devices that also have contraceptive implications, then they become much easier to understand. For example, those designed to correct a displacement included a splint to press the uterus forward or backward, which also served the same function as a modern IUD, and rings designed to cover the entrance to the uterus, many of which had domes fitted over them and thus acted in the same way as a modern diaphragm or cap. Other pessaries were developed to provide a roof to the vagina to hold a prolapse in place, and this also acted as a contraceptive. In retrospect, in fact, it seems that many of the so-called female complaints of the past, which led physicians and surgeons to prescribe such devices, were efforts to find some socially acceptable way of avoiding pregnancy. Historians can easily trace the development of such pessaries in the United States because they could be patented and advertised while devices claiming to have contraceptive value were not protected until well into the twentieth century.

It is not known who first realized that some pessaries had contraceptive potential, but it is clear that many women who wore them had neither a prolapsed uterus nor a uterine displacement. One of the earliest medical references to the contraceptive value of a pessary was by Friedrich Adolph Wilde, a German who urged women who wanted to avoid becoming pregnant to be fitted with a pessary made of unvulcanized India rubber (or *kautchuk* in German). His pessary was individually fitted. Wilde first took a wax impression of the cervix and then, using it as a pattern, designed a hard rubber pessary that would snugly cover the os or entrance into the cervix.[3] Today Wilde's device would be called a cervical cap.

Two developments that took place in the last part of the nineteenth century made the barrier types of contraceptive much more effective. One was the discovery of a method of making liquid latex (in 1853) and the other was the development of spermicides, which, when combined with the barrier methods, made a highly effective contraceptive. Chapter 6 will deal more specifically with spermicides, but it is important to emphasize that the barrier methods are most effective when combined with spermicides.

It did not take long for the discovery of latex to be applied to contraceptive methods.[4] Several diaphragm-like pessaries were patented in the nineteenth century, but the one most used was developed by Dr. C. Hasse of Flensburgh in Germany, who used the pseudonym of Wilhelm P. J. Mensinga. He utilized a latex cover for the top of the vagina held in place above the pubic bone by a coiled spring similar to that used in wind-up spring alarm clocks.[5] A student of Hasse (Mensinga), Dr. Aletta Jacobs, opened a contraceptive clinic in the Netherlands using the Mensinga diaphragm and its use spread rapidly. Margaret Sanger, who visited the Netherlands many years later, was shown some fourteen sizes of diaphragms designed to fit vaginal canals of differing sizes and proportions. Comstock laws prevented the mass importation of the Mensinga diaphragm into the United States before Sanger's demonstrations, although many were smuggled in. It was not until the 1920s, when the Holland-Rantos Company began manufacturing diaphragms, that they became readily available.[6] At the very outset, quality control was more effective than for many other kinds of contraceptive devices because, as a pessary, even though its primary use was as a contraceptive, it could be given patent protection.

Prior to the development of IUDs and oral contraceptives, the diaphragm, when combined with spermicidal jelly, was probably the most widely used contraceptive in the United States. The difficulty with the diaphragm is the same as with many other methods of contraception: it requires a high level of motivation. Traditionally it proved to be most effective among middle- and upper-class women. Since the diaphragm with spermicide does not interfere with any of the body's physiological functions, it is also extremely safe. The drop-off in its popularity was most noticeable during the 1960s and early 1970s when oral contraceptives appeared on the market. For example, 64 percent of the women attending Planned Parenthood clinics in 1961 chose the diaphragm compared to only 4 percent in 1973.[7] Since then the rate has increased slightly, and the combination of diaphragm and spermicide is still the contraceptive choice for many women.

DIAPHRAGMS

Types

There are several types of diaphragms on the market, but in the United States three are dominant: coil spring, flat spring, and the arcing spring or Findlay.

1. The *coil spring* has traditionally been the most common in the United States. It contains a round, spiral-coiled metal wire in the rim, encircled with rubber. It is suitable for the average woman who has strong vaginal muscles, a deep arch behind the *symphysis pubis* (pubic bone), no displacement of the uterus, and a normal size and contour of the vagina. It can be folded by compressing the rim and easily inserted or removed either by hand or with a plastic inserter.

2. The *flat spring* is the original Mensinga diaphragm in which the metal spring is more delicate than the coiled spring. It can be used by many of the same women who use the coiled spring types but it is particularly suitable for a woman who has a shallow arch behind the pubic bone. It is most useful for a woman who has never had a child.

DIAPHRAGM

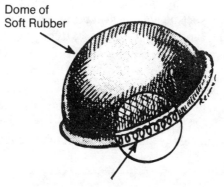

Dome of Soft Rubber

Spring (coil-spring type)

From Our Bodies, Ourselves, 1979. Illustration reproduced by permission of the Boston Women's Health Book Collective.

3. The *arcing spring* diaphragm has a double spring in the rim, which produces strong pressure against the vaginal walls. It is appropriately named because it forms an arc when the rim is compressed. It is most suitable for a woman with poor vaginal muscle tone, with a moderate cystocele (a bulging of the urinary bladder into the vagina), a rectocele (a bulging of the rectum into the vagina), or a mild uterine prolapse. Because the rim exerts such strong pressure against the vaginal walls, it has to be fitted with great care in order to avoid excessive pressure either on the vaginal wall or on the urethra, which would cause pain or difficulty in urinating. Since the arcing-spring diaphragm tends to flip into the correct position inside the vagina, it is next to impossible to insert it improperly. This makes it popular with many health care providers.[8]

Fitting

Since the effectiveness of the diaphragm, regardless of type, depends upon a good fit, a prescription is required for purchase. It requires a knowledgeable professional to select the correct size and type. Physicians, nurse practitioners, nurse midwives, and physicians' assistants are all licensed to do this. A diaphragm that is too small may slip out of place and expose the cervix, while one that is too large may buckle. Ideally, the fitter chooses the largest size diaphragm that fits evenly in the vaginal canal without the woman being aware of its presence.

Periodic checkups also might be needed to see if the diaphragm still fits. This is particularly true if there is a weight gain or loss of fifteen or more pounds, if pelvic surgery takes place, if there has been a delivery or a second trimester abortion, or if there was great tension during the initial fitting. The last of these might be a problem for a woman who is frightened or upset during the fitting since such tension can cause the vaginal muscles to tighten, resulting in the selection of a smaller diaphragm than should have been the case.

Procedures

Before insertion, a small amount of contraceptive jelly is put in the bowl of the diaphragm and a little is also applied around the edge of the rim with the fingertip. The opposite sides of the rim are then

INSERTING A DIAPHRAGM

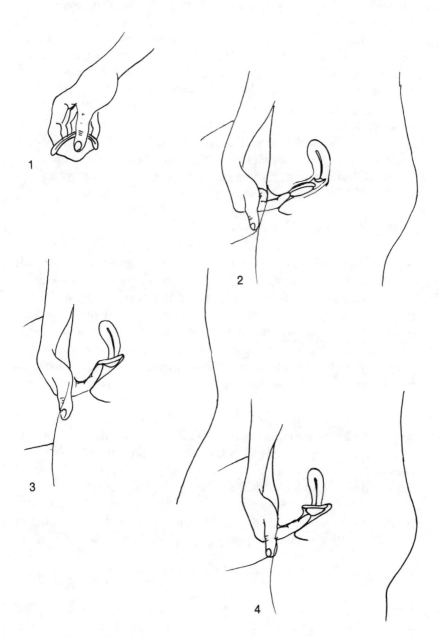

Illustration by Steven Bullough

compressed together so the diaphragm folds in the middle and the now-flattened shape is inserted into the vagina, usually with the bowl shape (containing the spermicide) against the cervix (although the dome can be used just as well if there is spermicide on the dome). Once inserted, the flexible rim allows the diaphragm to resume its original molded shape. Insertion is usually with the fingers although some women prefer to use an inserter. After it is inserted, the diaphragm should be checked to see that it is properly placed, fitting securely and comfortably between the rear wall of the vagina and the upper edge of the pubic bone. The cervix should be palpated—it feels like the end of a nose—to see that it is well covered by the rubber. In the proper position, the diaphragm completely covers the cervix and holds the contraceptive jelly tightly cupped over the entrance to the womb, thus providing both a mechanical and chemical barrier to the entry of sperm.

Insertion can be done from a number of different positions: sitting on the edge of a chair or toilet; lying flat on one's back with knees bent; squatting; or propping up one leg on the seat of a chair, the edge of a bathtub, or other objects of similar height. The diaphragm can be inserted up to six hours before intercourse, but if more than two hours elapse before coitus, the application of additional spermicide is recommended. If there is more than one act of intercourse, there should also be a second application of spermicidal jelly without removing the diaphragm. In fact, it should not be removed for six to eight hours after intercourse to ensure that the spermicide has worked. However, in no case should the diaphragm be kept in much longer than this since research suggests that there is a possibility of toxic shock syndrome occurring if it is left in for twenty-four hours or more. It is recommended that no douching take place while the diaphragm is in the vagina since this might dilute the spermicide.

Before inserting the diaphragm, it should be inspected for holes or tears, either visually by holding it up to the light or by placing water inside the dome to see if drops are collected underneath. If the rubber is puckered, it should not be used. A diaphragm that is properly cared for should last a year or two.

Effectiveness

The failure rate of diaphragms is calculated at somewhat less than
10 per 100 woman-years of use. This means that for every 100 women
using the diaphragm with spermicide for one year, less than 10 will
become pregnant. Failures are most likely to occur among new users
of the device. More experienced users tend to have lower failure rates;
some would claim no more than two or three per 100 woman-years
of use.

Advantages

Women using the diaphragm need only concern themselves with being protected at those times when they anticipate having intercourse.
The diaphragm and spermicidal jelly can be inserted just before intercourse or a couple of hours earlier. If the diaphragm is properly
positioned, the woman should not feel it—and neither, for that matter, should her partner. Women using this method need not get up
after intercourse to douche. The diaphragm may be left in place for
up to twelve hours at any one time, even including the onset of the
menses. It should be washed with soap and water, dried, and stored
in the plastic container designed to hold it until it is used again. The
diaphragm need not be replaced after every use; however, a new one
should be purchased every two years. Cost is minimal once the diaphragm has been fitted, and is primarily limited to the expense of
purchasing contraceptive jelly. Biologically, the diaphragm is one of
the safest contraceptives.

Side Effects

Generally, use of the diaphragm is free of serious side effects, although some women do have an allergic reaction to rubber (in such
cases, a plastic diaphragm is recommended), vaginal irritation (relieved by changing brands of spermicide), or infection (this last, as
indicated, is most likely to occur if the diaphragm is worn for more
than twenty-four hours). A diaphragm that is too large might also
cause some pain. Frequent bouts of cystitis, however, would suggest
that the woman should seek some other contraceptive since the pressure of the diaphragm on the bladder can further irritate both the

bladder and the urethra. This is because the bladder is separated from the vagina by only a thin wall of soft tissue.

Disadvantages

The diaphragm is a prescription item that must be fitted by a licensed health care provider. It requires some practice in learning how to insert and use the device, and the learning procedure is embarrassing for many women. As the user becomes expert, however, the embarrassment subsides. Replacing a diaphragm requires a prescription. Though this provision was enacted to ensure that women get a proper fit each time, it does require a visit to one's medical provider or to a suitably staffed clinic. The diaphragm must be used whenever intercourse takes place, so the user must either plan ahead for sex or interrupt love play to insert the diaphragm and jelly.

THE CERVICAL CAP

The cervical cap is a small thimble-shaped cup that only blocks the cervix and not the entire upper part of the vaginal canal as does the diaphragm. It was widely used at the beginning of the twentieth century when it was in competition with the diaphragm. It then fell into disfavor in the United States (though not in Great Britain), in part because it took longer to fit properly and seemed more complicated for the average consumer than the diaphragm. As a result, most contraceptive clinics prescribed the diaphragm. Once fitted, however, the cervical cap is held in place by suction, avoiding the pressure of the diaphragm, which was a source of discomfort for a few users.

Even though the cap was strongly advocated by some feminist health organizations in the 1970s, it ran into trouble in 1979 as a result of the Medical Device Amendment Act of 1976. This act marked the full-scale entry of the government into the contraceptive field, since before this there had been a lack of standards not only for various forms of contraceptives, but for the many new medical technologies entering the market in ever-increasing numbers. The government's intent was not to ban the cervical cap. In fact, the law only stipulated that manufacturers of all medical devices on the market before 1976 had to provide the Food and Drug Administration (FDA) with data on safety and efficacy as well as proof that the device had been marketed in the United States before that year. When Lamberts Ltd., the British manufacturer of the cap, for some reason (probably cost) failed to provide the needed information, the FDA had no alternative but to place the cap on its Class III list of devices—those that represent a significant risk to the user—and order the seizure of all cap shipments entering the country. Though the cap was not widely used in the United States, there were many strong advocates who urged that the ban be lifted. Tests were run, data gathered, and on May 23, 1988, the FDA announced its approval of one type of cap, the Prentif cavity-rim cervical cap for general use, and once again made this device available to those who prefer it.[9]

The Prentif cavity-rim cervical cap is made of a soft, pliable latex and is about half the size of the diaphragm. It is available in four sizes, with inside diameters of 22, 25, 28, and 31mm. It is the most commonly used in the United States and the first to be approved under the new regulations.

CERVICAL CAPS

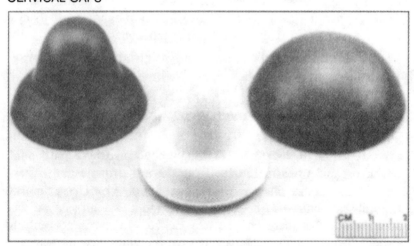

There are three types of cervical cap: the Vimule (left); the Prentif cavity-rim (center); and the Dumas, or vault cap (right). The Prentif cap is the most widely used.

Photograph reproduced courtesy of Population Reports.

Fitting

Like the diaphragm, the cervical cap must be fitted. The rim of the cap must approximate the circumference of the base of the cervix and fit evenly around that area without touching the cervical os. To position it, the health care provider inserts a vaginal speculum in order to expose the cervix and then selects a cap of the right size.[10]

Use

Before insertion, spermicidal jelly should be put into the cap until it is about one-third full. Too much jelly makes it difficult to obtain the necessary suction. The cap is inserted while the woman is in either a squatting or half-reclining position. The cap is held dome down between the thumb and forefinger, compressing the rim, and then, separating the labia with the fingers of the other hand, the cap is pushed along the posterior wall of the vaginal canal as far as it will go. Using the forefinger, the rim is pressed around the cervix until the dome covers the cervical os and the tip of the cervix can be felt under the dome, similar to the feel of the cervix through the diaphragm. The cap should remain in place a minimum of six to eight hours following intercourse, and the user should not douche until it is removed at that time. Unlike the diaphragm, the cap can be left in for two or three days at a time. It is removed by tilting the rim away from the cervix, thus breaking the suction. The index or middle finger can then hook under the rim and withdraw the cap. It is also possible to remove the dome by grasping it between the index and middle finger and pulling downward.[11]

Advantages

The demand for the return of the cap to the U.S. market was due largely to the fact that some women find it more comfortable and less messy than the diaphragm. Though technically the cap was still available after the ban, it was classified as an investigative device: physicians and clinics dispensing it had to carry out FDA-approved studies of safety and efficacy, and only a few clinics, mainly in large cities, did such studies. Plastic caps have several advantages over

INSERTING A CERVICAL CAP

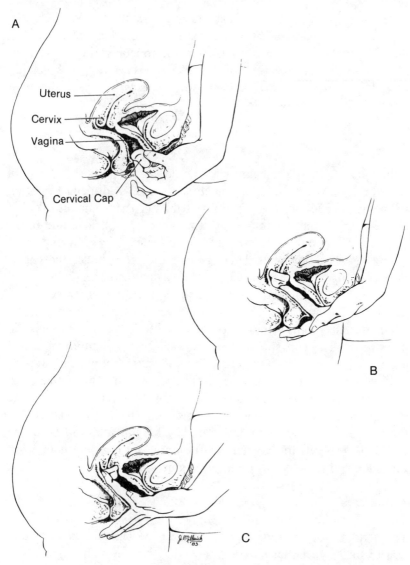

To insert a cervical cap, a woman compresses it and pushes it into the vagina as far as it will go (A). Then she checks that the cap is in position over the cervix (B). To remove it, she hooks her finger over the cap rim, dislodges it from the cervix, and pulls it out (C).

Illustration reproduced courtesy of Population Reports.

rubber-based contraceptives in that they do not react to acidic vaginal fluids and are not weakened or destroyed by animal or vegetable oils and thus may be used with spermicides that have an oil base. Failure rates seem to be similar to those of the diaphragm, although improper fitting, causing the cap to be dislodged, is more likely than among diaphragm users.[12] The cap has the advantage, over the diaphragm, of not creating pressure on the bladder, and it also does not block the stimulation of the anterior vaginal wall, which some researchers have claimed is the site of the Gräfenberg or "G" spot, a particularly sensitive area of sexual pleasure for some women.[13]

Side Effects

Like the diaphragm, the cap is free of side effects. It should not, however, be worn by a woman with a history of abnormal Pap smears. Present regulations for its use advise that a Pap smear be performed after three months' use to make certain that there is not a link between its use and abnormal Pap smears. Some users of the cap have complained of vaginal odor and partner discomfort. Vaginal odor can be avoided if the cap is removed within 48 to 72 hours after insertion. The cap is not suitable for every woman, particularly those whose cervixes are too short, too long, or have an irregular shape. Like any barrier method, the cervical cap relies heavily on user persistence and technique. Those who use it have to feel comfortable with and about their own anatomy for it to be effective.

Other Caps

Two other caps, the vault (or Dumas) cap and the Vimule cap, which differ slightly from the cervical cap, are available although not necessarily in the United States. The vault or Dumas cap is made of rubber or plastic and shaped like a circular bowl with a thick rim and thin center. It clings by suction to the vault or roof of the vagina, following the contour of the cervix. It is useful for the woman who cannot accommodate a diaphragm because of poor muscle tone, and for the woman who cannot use the Prentif cervical cap because her cervix is either too long or too short. The Dumas cap is available in five sizes ranging from 50 to 75 mm., and while the diameters are larger than the Prentif cavity-rim cup, this is because it, like the

THE SPONGE

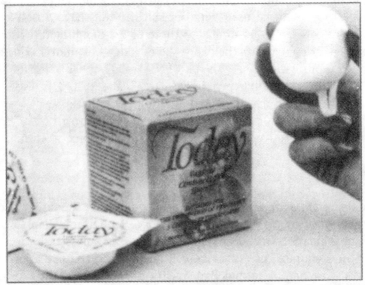

The 24-hour contraceptive sponge is an over-the-counter product that acts as both a chemical and physical barrier to sperm. Although effectiveness varies among study groups, proponents of the sponge stress that the product is safe and convenient.
Photograph reproduced courtesy of Population Reports.

Vimule cap, covers the cervix and part of the upper vaginal vault while the Prentif only covers the cervix. The Vimule cap is a longer bell-shaped cap made of thick rubber or plastic with a deep dome. It fits around the cervix but has a flanged rim that permits it to be pressed more firmly onto the roof of the vagina. It is useful for a woman who has poor vaginal muscle tone, a cystocele, or a longer than average cervix. It is available in three sizes: 42, 48, and 54 mm.[13]

THE SPONGE

Though the use of a sponge is an old method of contraception, the modern sponge only dates from the mid-1970s when the U.S. government-funded Program for Applied Research on Fertility Regulation supported research at the University of Arizona into the use of the sponge. The first sponge, made mostly of collagen, a fibrous animal protein, was intended to be reusable. Containing no spermicide, it was supposed to block the cervix and absorb ejaculate. Though initial acceptability was encouraging, preliminary studies indicated a high failure rate, and the project was dropped. Working independently, Bruce Vorhauer, founder of VLI Corporation of California, introduced a polyurethane sponge impregnated with non-oxynol-9, a spermicide. The sponges, with different percentages of the spermicide, were tested in Mexico City in 1977. All of the early sponges were supposed to be reusable for several months, although they were to be washed out periodically. Failure rates in the Mexico City experiment were quite high because the women apparently washed their sponges so vigorously that most of the spermicide was washed away. With modifications in size, shape, and color, and with a standardized 30 percent solution of nonoxynol-9, the sponge was again tested for multiple use in a variety of countries. This time the washing was limited to ten times. Again there were problems with the washing of the sponge; it was finally decided that the best version of the sponge was a single use, disposable product. The sponge also was changed to a mushroom cap shape so that it took up less space in the vagina and fitted more snugly against the cervix. The current sponge is designed to fit in the upper vagina with the concave side covering the cervix. In this form and under the trademark *Today,* it has been sold in the United States since July 1983. The sponge can be worn for up to twenty-four hours and for any number of acts of intercourse during that time, and perhaps most importantly, it can be purchased over the counter.

Effectiveness

Though the sponge is not as effective as the diaphragm or cap plus spermicide, it is more effective for some women than others. Studies suggest that women who have had children (parous women), married women, and/or older women may be at a greater risk of accidental pregnancy when using the sponge than those who have not had children, who are unmarried, and who are younger. Among married women, sponge users had a pregnancy rate of 24.2 per 100 woman-years while diaphragm users in the same group had a rate of 6.2. Among single women, both diaphragm and sponge users had a rate of about 14 per 100 woman-years.[14] Advocates of the sponge believed the high failure rate among parous women could be lowered by the use of a larger sponge. Research is still continuing, but at this point it seems clear that the sponge is not as effective as the diaphragm or cap and spermicide, particularly for the older woman.

Use

After removing the sponge from its air-tight pack, it should be held in one hand with the "dimple" side up and the loop (used to remove it) dangling down. The sponge at this juncture should feel slightly moist. Wet it more with a small amount of water but not more than two tablespoons. The sponge should then be squeezed gently to remove excess water until it feels moist and soggy but not dripping wet. Fold the side of the sponge upward with a finger along each side to support it. The sponge should look long and narrow. It is imperative that the string loop dangles underneath the sponge from one end of the fold to the other. With the woman in a squatting position, her legs spread apart, the sponge is inserted by using the free hand to part the lips of the vagina. As is the case with inserting a diaphragm or cervical cap, it is also possible to implant the sponge while standing with one foot on a chair or toilet seat, sitting cross-legged, or by lying down, whichever position is most comfortable. The sponge is then slid into the opening of the vagina as far as the fingers will go. As the sponge slides through the fingers, the fingers are used to push it up into the vagina as far as it will go. Care should be taken not to puncture it with a fingernail. The position of the sponge should be checked by sliding a finger around its edge to make sure that the cervix is not exposed and that the loop can be felt.

Side Effects

The most commonly documented side effects of the contraceptive sponge are allergic-type reactions and vaginal irritations. Some users complain of such vaginal discomfort as soreness, itching, dryness, and stinging. Some experts have expressed fear about the possible dangers of toxic shock syndrome for users. Although this is a possibility, there is some evidence that the spermicides present in most barrier contraceptives protect against the syndrome.[15] To be on the safe side, the sponge should be removed within twenty-four hours of insertion.[16]

Advantages

The sponge provides protection for up to twenty-four hours regardless of the frequency of coitus, and it requires no waiting after insertion. The sponge is easy to use, less messy than spermicides, and it does not require a prescription for purchase.

Disadvantages

Women who object to inserting an object into the vagina and later removing it will find the contraceptive sponge unsatisfactory. Some women are more uncomfortable with it than with the diaphragm or cervical cap; and the sponge is not as effective for some groups as the diaphragm or cap combined with spermicide, particularly older women or those who have experienced pregnancy.

CONCLUSION

The barrier contraceptives provide another alternative. Two of the three, diaphragms and cervical caps, have the disadvantage that they are (1) available only by prescription, and (2) must be fitted by a health care provider. Both of these methods are highly effective provided they are combined with contraceptive jelly. The third method, the sponge, is not as effective, at least for some groups, as the other two, but it has the advantage of being sold over the counter. All three methods require women to be able to insert and withdraw material from their vaginas, something that some women find distasteful or embarrassing. Each method also requires advance planning since insertion has to take place before intercourse. There is also still another barrier contraceptive, the condom, but since it depends upon the male for its effectiveness, this will be discussed in chapter 8.

NOTES

1. B. E. Finch, "Balls, Feathers and Caps," in B. E. Finch and H. Green, eds., *Contraception Through the Ages* (Springfield, Ill.: Charles C. Thomas, 1963), pp. 38–45, and N. E. Himes, *Medical History of Contraception* (reprinted New York: Schocken Books, 1970).

2. See also "The Diaphragm and Other Intravaginal Barriers: A Review," a report prepared by Judith Wortman, *Population Reports*, Series H, Number 4 (January 1976).

3. F. A. Wilde, *Das weibliche Gebär-unvermögen* (Berlin, 1838).

4. Vern L. Bullough, "A Brief Note on Rubber Technology and Contraception: The Diaphragm and the Condom," *Technology and Culture* 22 (January 1981): 104–11.

5. W. P. J. Mensinga, *Über facultative Sterilität*, 2 vols., 2d ed. (Neuweid and Leipzig, 1885).

6. D. M. Kennedy, *Birth Control in America: The Career of Margaret Sanger* (New Haven: Yale University Press, 1970).

7. B. Weidiger, "Diaphragms: A New Look at the Old Standby," *MS.* 4 (August 1975): 101–104.

8. R. A. Hatcher, F. Guest, F. Stewart, G. K. Stewart, J. Trussel, S. C. Bowen, and W. Cates, *Contraceptive Technology 1988–1989*, 14th rev. ed. (New York: Irvington Publishers, Inc., 1988).

9. Michael Klitsch, "FDA Approval Ends Cervical Cap's Marathon," *Family Planning Perspectives* 20 (May/June 1988): 137–38.

10. Hans Lehfeldt, "Cervical Cap," in Mary S. Calderone, *Manual of Family Planning and Contraceptive Practice* (Baltimore: Williams and Wilkins, 1970), pp. 368–75.

11. J. Peel and M. Potts, "Diaphragms and Caps," in Peel and Potts, eds., *Textbook of Contraceptive Practice* (Cambridge: Cambridge University Press, 1969), pp. 62–73; Planned Parenthood Federation of America, Medical Committee, *Methods of Birth Control in the United States* (New York: Planned Parenthood Federation of America, 1972), and C. Tietze, H. Lehfeldt, and H. G. Liebmann, "The Effectiveness of the Cervical Cap as a Contraceptive Method," *American Journal of Obstetrics and Gynecology* 66 (October 1953), 904–908,.

12. M. Klitsch, "FDA Approval Ends Cervical Caps Marathon," pp. 61–73; R. Caen, "The Cervical Cap as a Barrier Contraceptive," *Contraception* 33 (May 1986): 487–96.

13. A. K. Ladas, B. Whipple, and J. D. Perry, *The G Spot and Other Recent Discoveries About Human Sexuality* (New York: Holt, Rinehart, and Winston, 1982).

14. Peel and Potts, "Diaphragms and Caps." See also H. Wright, *Contraceptive Technique* (London: J. and A. Churchill, 1968), and J. A. Loraine, "Other Methods of Birth Control," in J. A. Loraine, ed., *Sex and the Population Crisis* (London: William Heinemann, 1970), pp. 54–70.

15. D. A., Edelman, *Development and Testing of Vaginal Contraceptives: Final Report* (Research Triangle Park, N.C.: Family Health International, 1983) (NIH Contract No. NO1-HD-1-2800). Cited in

"New Developments in Contraception," *Population Reports*, Series H, Number 7 (January-February 1984): Vol. 12, Number 1.

16. J. D. Shelton and J. E. Higgins, "Contraception and Toxic-Shock Syndrome: A Reanalysis," *Contraception* 24 (December 1981): 631–34.

4

Oral Contraceptives

Oral contraceptives are synthetic hormones that prevent pregnancy. They were first approved by the federal Food and Drug Administration (FDA) in 1960. Though FDA approval was not then necessary for devices, it was for pharmaceuticals, and so the pill, in effect, was the first contraceptive approved by the U.S. government. This marked a breakthrough in what had previously been governmental inaction in the field of contraception. The research that resulted in the pill had started out as an effort to control menstrual pain some three decades earlier. After the hormone progesterone was isolated, it was found as early as 1936 that daily injections of it prevented the estrus cycle in rats. Further research with humans demonstrated that a combination of both estrogen and progesterone was more effective in preventing ovulation and dysmenorrhea than either hormone alone. Other researchers soon realized the important potential of these findings for birth control as well as for the control of menstrual pain.[1]

Before additional experiments could be done on a large scale, it was necessary to develop synthetic hormones; those extracted from animals were not only expensive but both the progesterone and estrogen derived from animals tended to be destroyed by enzymes in the human body. It was at this point that the pharmaceutical industry entered the picture. A researcher named Carl Djerassi, at the Syntex Laboratories in Mexico City, converted a substance found in the Mexican yam into a synthetic progestin (the term now applied to all progesterone-like substances). Using this knowledge other synthetic substances could be developed, including synthetic estrogen. The eventual result was a pill that combined the two drugs.

Gregory Pincus and his colleagues working at the Worcester Foundation for Experimental Biology in Massachusetts moved the experiments from the laboratory to the field and tested the anovulatory drugs in a series of small-scale studies on women. When this research was successful, they planned and carried out a full-scale study in Puerto Rico. A group of 265 women were given pills containing 10 milligrams (mg.) of progestin and varying amounts of estrogen. Before the study the rate of pregnancy among the women in the sample was 63 per 100 years of marriage (a very high rate of pregnancy). The results were astonishing. No woman who took the pill every day for a 20-day cycle each month became pregnant during the study, which lasted almost two years.[2,3] However, some women dropped out of the study, reporting very uncomfortable side effects including nausea, dizziness, vomiting, and pelvic pain. We now know that these side effects are related to the high doses of estrogen and progestin in those early pills. This was also true of those persons who took Enovid, the first pill marketed for general use in 1960. It included 10 mg. of progestin and 150 micrograms (mcg.) of estrogen, and the side effects were a problem for many women then as well. The history of the development of the oral contraceptives has been one of gradually decreasing doses to lessen the side effects.

The development of oral contraceptives marked the beginning of a new era for women, finally putting an end to the long-held belief that biology was destiny, thereby giving women more effective control over their physiological processes. Some testimony to the importance of oral contraceptives in the lives of women is the fact that the term "the pill" has been applied to them rather than to any of the many thousands of other pills on the market.

THE FUNCTION OF ORAL CONTRACEPTIVES

Oral contraceptives work by interfering with the hormonal system, thus controlling ovulation and related reproductive functions. As indicated earlier, the normal menstrual cycle is regulated by an area in the brain called the hypothalamus, which works through the pituitary to regulate ovarian function. The pituitary gland secretes two hormones: the follicle-stimulating hormone (FSH), which signals the follicle in the ovary to develop, and the luteinizing hormone (LH), which signals the follicle to release the egg (ovum). These two hormones travel through the bloodstream to reach the ovary.

In response to the FSH an ovarian follicle (or egg sac) develops in the ovary. This follicle releases the hormone estrogen while the egg is ripening. During the first few days of the menstrual cycle the rate of release is slow, but as the follicle develops the supply of estrogen increases until just before the time for ovulation when the estrogen level rises precipitously. When the estrogen secretions reach a certain level the hypothalamus sends a message to the pituitary gland, which in turn secretes LH, thereby triggering ovulation. After ovulation, the follicle that held the egg is renamed the corpus luteum (literally, yellow body). It produces both progesterone and estrogen. The progesterone stimulates the lining of the uterus (the endometrium) to expand, which allows the fertilized egg to be attached to it. If no fertilization takes place, both the estrogen and progesterone diminish and this build-up of the uterine lining is shed in a process known as menstruation.

Oral contraceptives, as synthetic hormones, replace and suppress the hormones that the body would have produced. Since they are administered in a constant dosage or in some other pattern differing from the normal cycle we described, a false signal is transmitted to the hypothalamus with the result that the signal triggering the ovulation process is not delivered. In addition, the hormones in the oral contraceptives alter the tubal transport system, change the cervical mucus, and alter the endometrium so that fertilization is not possible.[4]

TYPES OF PILLS

There are three types of oral contraceptives: combination pills, which include both estrogen and a progestin; triphasic pills, which include these same elements but in differing amounts during the cycle; and "mini-pills," which are low-dose progestins (without estrogen). The combination pills are the most popular and probably the most reliable. Current dosages usually include 1 mg. or less of progestin and 35 to 50 mcg. of estrogen. They come in a package designed to dispense one pill a day, and the days of the cycle are marked off to

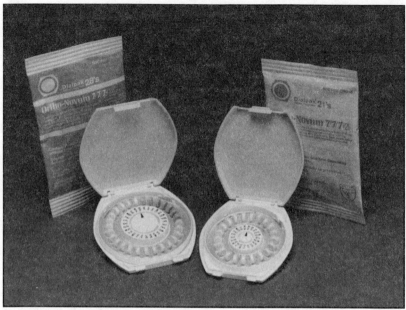

Photograph reproduced courtesy of Ortho Pharmaceutical Corporation, Raritan, N.J.

assist the user in keeping track of them. The pills are taken from the first day of the cycle (right after the menses end) to the twenty-first day. They are then discontinued until the end of the menstrual period. Some packages include an additional seven pills made of sugar or some inert substance, allowing users to take a tablet each day of the cycle. One effect of the pills is to make the menstrual cycles regular even for women who have never been regular.

The triphasic oral contraceptives came on the market in the 1980s, although in the 1960s there were sequential pills marketed for a time, which were later discontinued. These newer sequential tablets include three phases instead of two. They contain the same two ingredients (estrogen and progestin) as in the combination pills. Two of the popular preparations, Ortho-Novum 7/7/7 and Triphasil, start with a dose of progestin and gradually increase the amount during the cycle. Tri-Norinyl starts and ends with a low dose of progestin, with a higher dose in the middle.

These changes are aimed at trying to mimic the normal hormonal cycle in order to decrease side effects and increase user satisfaction. Skeptics also note the fact that the patents on many of the combination pills have run out so generic birth control pills are coming onto the market. The triphasics may represent a marketing effort that emphasizes new protected formulations.[5]

The mini-pills are low-dose, progestin-only contraceptives taken every day so that there is less chance of forgetting them. Though the absence of estrogen does cut down some of the side effects, these pills are rendered less effective in preventing pregnancy. The major side effect they do cause, namely bleeding, is distressing to many users. Mini-pills are now used primarily for lactating mothers (since estrogens are not good for the baby) as well as for those few women who find the estrogen-related side effects distressing.[6]

EFFECTIVENESS

When oral contraceptives are taken daily and regularly at about the same time, their level of effectiveness reaches 100 percent. In actual practice there are between 4 and 10 failures (pregnancies) per 100 woman-years, with most being caused by forgetting to take a pill or by delays in taking the pill. When such lapses happen, an alternative form of contraception (such as condom and sponge) should be used for the remainder of the month, along with the pill. Failure rates were lower when the dosages were higher, but as the doses came down to control for side effects, the failure rate for a forgotten pill or delay of more than four hours increased.

Oral contraceptives are the most popular form of birth control, being used by 31.1 percent of those Americans who use contraceptives. World-wide there are more than fifty million users.[7] There probably would be many millions more but the pill is not extensively used in Third World countries because population planning experts believe it takes more sophistication to use oral contraceptives than some alternatives, and the necessity for taking a pill every day at the same time is alien to the cultural patterns of many peoples. Nevertheless, the social impact of the pill is difficult to overestimate. For the first time a safe, reliable method of contraception was available to the average woman. The power that accrued to women when they could control conception was a major factor in the women's movement, in broadening the occupational opportunities for women, in the decline of prostitution, and in the increased prosperity of ordinary working families. As the pill and other effective contraceptives become more available to people in the Third World, the control of population will be a key element in their economic and political development.

SIDE EFFECTS

Cardiovascular risks are the most publicized problems as we grow older, and they are the complications that have caused most of the pill-related problems. For this reason, women with a history of stroke, coronary artery disease (angina or heart attack), embolisms, diabetes, thrombophlebitis, or other blood vessel problems should not take oral contraceptives, because it is these women who would be the most likely candidates for pill-induced strokes, heart attacks, or emboli.[8] The continued efforts of scientists and the pharmaceutical industry have been aimed at lessening the danger from these complications, and for the most part they have been successful. In the process, research has also identified those women most at risk to develop complications and it is women on these lists for whom the pill might be dangerous. First on the list are smokers since smoking damages the blood vessels. In fact, most of the women who have suffered serious complications are smokers. The other important risk factor is age. Thus a young woman who is a moderate smoker might take the pill, but a smoker who is past the age of thirty should not.[9, 10]

While cardiovascular problems constitute the major risk-factor related to oral contraceptives, some people worry more about breast cancer, probably due to media coverage of various recent studies. Most of the large-scale studies that assess the possible relationship between breast cancer and the pill have been completely negative.[11] However, in two recent studies certain sub-samples of the larger group were identified. Breast cancer was found to be more likely in those persons who started using the pill at a young age and continued it for many years than in women who did not use the pill.[12, 13] In addition, cervical cancer is somewhat more likely among pill users. On the other hand, oral contraceptives are apparently protective against uterine and ovarian cancer; pill users are less likely than the general public to develop these cancers.[14]

Minor side effects once associated with the pill have decreased over the years as lower dosages have become more common. Table 1 lists these side effects.

TABLE 1

COMMON SIDE EFFECTS ASSOCIATED WITH ORAL CONTRACEPTIVES

1. Weight gain and increased appetite
2. Edema (swelling)
3. Nausea
4. Vaginal discharge
5. Headaches
6. Breast changes
7. Chloasma (pigmentary skin discoloration)
8. Changes in menses or break-through bleeding
9. More or less libido (sex drive)
10. Rash
11. Sterility for several months after discontinuing the pill

---

Many of these side effects can be controlled by switching to a different pill that balances the estrogen-progestin content in a slightly different way. The process of determining the right pill is somewhat individualized, so the user needs to report her symptoms to a health care provider, who can often find a pill that better fits her needs. For an example, headaches during the premenstrual or menstrual phase of the cycle could be caused by too much progestin, while a headache during the remainder of the cycle might signal an estrogen excess in that particular woman. Similarly, increased appetite means a progestin excess, while nausea and edema relate to an estrogen excess.

A note of caution: Neither estrogen nor progestin should be taken during pregnancy. A couple who are planning a baby should stop the pill for at least one month and use an alternative contraceptive before attempting to conceive.

BENEFITS AND ADVANTAGES

Oral contraceptives also have some benefits for the health of the user. Since they were originally developed to cure primary dysmenorrhea (menstrual pain that is not related to some other cause), they are very effective in this regard. They are also very effective in decreasing the incidence of pelvic inflammatory disease, since the cervical mucus changes block bacteria from entering the uterus. Oral contraceptives lessen the pain of fibrocystic disease and probably lessen the cyst formation characteristic of the process. It is believed that the reduced pain is caused by lessening the fluctuations in the hormone levels. The pill also protects users against uterine and ovarian cancer, lowers the incidence of endometriosis, reduces anemia, and may also reduce the incidence of rheumatoid arthritis.[15]

NOTES

1. J. Bennett, *Chemical Contraception* (New York: Columbia University Press, 1974).

2. G. Pincus, J. Rock, C-R. Garcia, E. Rice-Wray, M. Paniagua, and I. Rodriguez, "Fertility Control with Oral Medication," reprinted in *Benchmark Papers in Human Physiology: Contraception*, edited by L. L. Langley (Stroudsburg, Penn.: Dowden, Hutchinson & Ross), pp. 413–26.

3. G. Pincus, *The Control of Fertility* (New York: Academic Press, 1965).

4. L. Martin, *The Health Care of Women* (Philadelphia: J. P. Lippincott, 1978).

5. R. A. Hatcher, F. Guest, F. Stewart, G. K. Stewart, J. Trussell, S. C. Bowen, and W. Cates, *Contraceptive Technology, 1988-1989*, 14th rev. ed. (New York: Irvington Publishers, Inc., 1988) pp. 194–250.

6. "Mini-pill—A Limited Alternative for Certain Women," *Population Reports*, Oral Contraceptives, Series A, Number 3 (September 1975): A53–A67.

7. N. B. Attico, "Contraception Update," *The IHS Primary Care Provider* 14 (July 1989): 77–85.

8. "Oral Contraceptives in the 1980s," *Population Reports*, Series A, Number 6 (May-June 1982): Vol. 10, No. 3.

9. L. C. Jones, "Oral Contraceptives," *Nursing Drug Reference: A Practitioner's Guide*, edited by M. Edmunds (Bowie, Md.: Brady Communications Co., Inc., 1985), pp. 849–957.

10. S. Stone, "Assessing Oral Contraceptive Risks," *Medical Aspects of Human Sexuality* (April 1989): 112–21.

11. The Centers for Disease Control Cancer and Steroid Hormone Study, "Long-term Oral Contraceptive Use and the Risk of Breast Cancer," *Journal of the American Medical Association* 249 (March 25, 1983): 1591–95.

12. C. R. Kay and P. C. Hannaford, "Breast Cancer and the Pill— A Further Report from the Royal College of General Practitioners' Oral Contraceptive Study," *British Journal on Cancer* 58 (1988): 675–80.

13. B. B. Standel, S. Lai, J. J. Schlesselman, and P. Murray, "Oral Contraceptives and Premenopausal Breast Cancer in Nulliparous Women," *Contraception* 38 (September 1988): 287–99.

14. D. R. Mishell, "Medical Progress: Contraception," *New England Journal of Medicine* 320 (1989): 777–87.

15. N. B. Attico, "Contraception Update," pp. 77–85.

5

Intrauterine Devices (IUDs)

Using an intrauterine device (IUD) is many times safer than pregnancy and more effective in preventing pregnancy than oral contraceptives, condoms, spermicides, barrier methods, or natural family planning. The current generation of IUDs is safe for most women and about 99 percent effective over one year of use. Not all women should use IUDs, however, and they have not always been as safe as they now are.

As with most contraceptives, IUDs have a long history. Most of the early manifestations, however, were not technically IUDs but stem pessaries, since most of the devices were placed in the vagina with a stem extending through the cervical opening into the uterus. While nominally inserted to correct uterine positions, they also induced abortions as well as prevented pregnancies. Drawings of these devices, many of which were patented, would indicate that they also often made intercourse difficult.

In the twentieth century several German physicians experimented with IUDs made of silkworm gut either for use as a true IUD or as a stem pessary. By this time, however, the whole process of infection was well understood, and only a few physicians prescribed such devices; most feared they would cause pelvic infection. Before the discovery of antibiotics such infections were invariably fatal. The first IUD to be widely used was a ring of gut and silver wire developed by Ernst Gräfenberg, a German gynecologist and sex researcher, which became popular in Germany in the late 1920s.[1] In 1934, Tenrei Ota of Japan introduced gold and gold-plated silver intrauterine rings, which he claimed were more effective than Gräfenberg's device.[2] Though there was initial enthusiasm for these devices, both quickly ran into difficulty. The Japanese government for a time prohibited the use of Ota's device, while Gräfenberg abandoned his ring because of opposition by European physicians. Again the opposition came because of fear of uterine infection.

As the new antibiotics finally overcame such fears, several physicians began to experiment with IUDs. The major turning point occurred at an international conference on IUDs held in New York City in 1962 under the auspices of the Population Council. At the meeting physicians from the United States, Israel, Germany, and elsewhere reported on their favorable experiences with IUDs.[3] Also important in encouraging further research was the development of polyethylene, a biologically inert plastic that could be molded into any desired configuration. It was flexible (thus easily inserted into the uterus) and could spring back to its predetermined shape.

One of the key figures in the development of a safe, functional IUD and in bringing about an attitude change regarding its use was Jack Lippes, a gynecologist from Buffalo, New York. Influenced by reports of the successful use of IUDs (19,000 using the Ota ring in Japan and 866 women using the Gräfenberg ring in Israel), Lippes began to use the Gräfenberg ring—made from silkworm gut—on twenty of his own patients. Lippes soon ran into problems, primarily when trying to remove the device since it lacked a tail and required him to use an instrument similar to a crochet hook for retrieval. Lippes found this a difficult procedure and began experimenting with the Ota ring, to which he attached a string that dangled through the cervix. Although this facilitated removal, in about 20 percent of his cases the Ota ring would rotate and wind the string up into the uterine cavity.[4] As he continued his experiments, Lippes tried making a polyethylene loop with a monofilament thread of the same material hanging from it. Initially this caused difficulty because the thread was hard to see in the vagina, but after dying the thread blue he found he could see it and thus easily remove the IUD. The existence of the blue thread also allowed women to check that the device was still in place. Though there were other competitors such as the Margulies Spiral and the Binberg Bows, the Lippes Loop became the best known and most widely used device in developing countries outside of China. The loops are available in four types, from the

WIDELY USED INTRAUTERINE DEVICES
CHARACTERISTICS AND DISTRIBUTION

Reproduced courtesy of Population Reports.

TCu-380A, TCu-380Ag, and TCu-380 Slimline (TCu-380S)

Description: Polyethylene with barium sulfate added for visibility on x-rays. 314 mm^2 copper wire on vertical stem; two 33 mm^2 solid copper sleeves on each transverse arm. The wire in the 380Ag has a silver core. On the 380S the copper sleeves are placed at the ends of the arms and recessed into the plastic.

Developers: Population Council (US) and Ortho Canada (TCu-380S)

Date first marketed: 1982 (TCu-380A)

Major distributors: TCu-380A—Finishing Enterprises, US; P.T. Kimia Farma, Indonesia (trial production); Produtos Medicos Ltda., Brazil; Gyno-Pharma, Inc., US (brand name Para-Gard; sales beginning 1988); TCu-380A and TCu-380S (brand name Gyne T Slimline)—Ortho Canada; TCu-380S—Cilag, France; TCu-

380Ag—Leiras Medica, Finland.

Length: 36 mm   **Width:** 32 mm

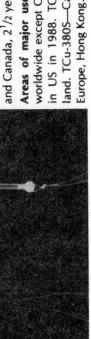

Strings: Two white (formerly blue)

Inserter type and diameter: Withdrawal; 4.4 mm (All use the same inserter tube, but TCu-380S arms fit completely in tube. With TCu-380A and Ag only the tips of the arms fit inside the tube.)

Approved lifespan: TCu-380A—US and UK, 4 years; various other European countries, 5 years. TCu-380Ag—Finland, 5 years. TCu-380S—various European countries and Canada, 2^1/2 years.

Areas of major use: TCu-380A—worldwide except China; available in US in 1988. TCu-380Ag—Finland. TCu-380S—Canada, Western Europe, Hong Kong.

TCu-200, TCu-200B, and TCu-200Ag

Description: Polyethylene with barium sulfate added for visibility on x-rays. 200 mm^2 copper wire wrapped around stem. The wire on the TCu-200Ag has a silver core. The TCu-200B (shown) has a ball at the tip of the stem; the TCu-200 does not.

Developers: Howard Tatum (US) and Jaime Zipper (Chile)

Date first marketed: 1972

Major distributors: TCu-200B—Finishing Enterprises, US, and Produtos Medicos Ltda., Brazil; TCu-200—Ortho Canada, and Leiras Medica, Finland; TCu-200Ag—Leiras Medica, Finland

Strings: Two; color varies

Inserter type and diameter: Withdrawal; 4.4 mm

Approved lifespan: US, 4 years; various European countries, 3 years

Areas of major use: Worldwide except China and US

Nova T

Description: Polyethylene with barium sulfate added for visibility on x-rays. 200 mm^2 copper wire with a silver core wrapped around the stem.

Developers: Outokumpu Oy (Finland)

Date first marketed: 1979

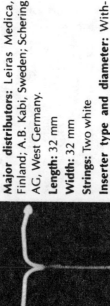

Major distributors: Leiras Medica, Finland; A.B. Kabi, Sweden; Schering AG, West Germany.

Length: 32 mm

Width: 32 mm

Strings: Two white

Inserter type and diameter: Withdrawal; 3.6 mm

Approved lifespan: Various European countries, 5 years

Areas of major use: Europe, Canada, Australia, New Zealand

Length: 36 mm   **Width:** 32 mm

Multiload-250 (MLCu-250) and 375 (MLCu-375)

Description: Polyethylene with two flexible arms with spurs. The MLCu-250 has 250 mm² copper wire on the stem and is available in 3 sizes (top, left to right)—Standard, Short, and Mini. The MLCu-375 has 375 mm² copper wire and is available in 3 sizes (bottom, left to right)—Standard, Short, and SL.

Developer: W.A.A. van Os (Netherlands)

Date first marketed: 1974

Distributors: Produced by Multilan AG, Switzerland; Biotechno, Brazil (for in-country distribution only); and P.T. Kimia Farma, Indonesia (trial production). Distributed through subsidiaries and agents of Organon, Netherlands, member of AKZO Pharma Group; Parke-Davis, Italy; Laboratoires CCD, France.

Length: Standard (250 and 375)—35 mm; 375SL—29 mm; 250 Short—24 mm; 250 Mini—24 mm

Width: Standard (250 and 375), 375SL, 250 Short—18 mm; 250 Mini—13 mm

Strings: Two black or colorless

Inserter type: Withdrawal (no plunger)

Insertion diameter: Standard (250 and 375), 375SL, and 250 Short—12 mm; Mini—9 mm. (Arms remain outside inserter tube.)

Approved lifespan: MLCu-250—most European countries, 3 years; MLCu-375—most European countries, 5 years.

Areas of major use: Europe; Australia; India; Indonesia and other Southeast Asian countries; New Zealand, Latin America.

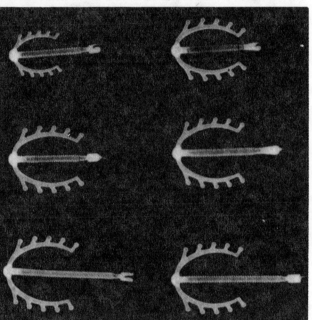

TCu-220C

Description: Polyethylene with barium sulfate added for visibility on x-rays. 220 mm^2 copper in seven copper sleeves—2 on the arms and 5 on the stem.

Developer: Population Council (US)

Date first marketed: 1980

Major distributors: Laboratorios Alpha, Mexico; Tianjin Medical Instrument Corporation, Factory No. 4, China (in-country distribution only).

Length: 36 mm   **Width:** 32 mm

Strings: Two

Inserter type and diameter: Withdrawal; 4.4 mm

Approved lifespan: Mexico, 3 years

Areas of major use: China, Mexico

Progestasert Intrauterine Progesterone Contraceptive System

Description: Ethylene vinyl acetate copolymer. Vertical stem contains a reservoir of 38 mg progesterone and barium sulfate (for visibility on x-rays) in silicone oil base. Releases 65 µg progesterone per day.

Developer: Alza Corp. (US)

Date first marketed: 1976

Distributors: Alza Corporation, US; Polcrome Ltd., UK; Theraplix Divison, Rhone Poulenc Santé, France.

Length: 36 mm   **Width:** 32 mm

Strings: Two blue-black

Inserter type and diameter: Withdrawal; 8 mm

Approved lifespan: US, one year; France,18 months.

Areas of major use: US, France

Lippes Loop

Description: Polyethylene with barium sulfate added for visibility on x-rays. Available in four sizes, designated A (left) through D (right).

Developer: Jack Lippes (US)

Date first marketed: 1962

Major distributors: Finishing Enterprises, US; P.T. Kimia Farma, Indonesia (in-country distribution only).

Length: A—26.2 mm; B—25.2 mm; C—27.5 mm; D—27.5 mm

Width: A—22.2 mm; B—27.4 mm; C—30.0 mm; D—30.0 mm

Strings: Two; A—blue, B—black, C—yellow, D—white

Inserter type and diameter: Push-out; 4.7 mm

Areas of major use: Developing countries except China

Chinese IUDs

Description: The most widely used IUD in China is the stringless single-coil stainless steel ring (1). The newly developed uterine cavity shaped steel ring is becoming widely used (2). It is replacing the Mahua ring, a double-coil stainless steel ring (3). Much less commonly used is the Shanghai V-200, made of silicone plastic on a wire frame with 200 mm^2 copper wire (4).

Size: The single-coil ring and the Mahua ring are produced in seven sizes ranging from 18 to 24 mm in diameter.

Strings: None on rings or on uterine-shaped device. Two black threads on Shanghai V-200.

Inserter type: Stainless steel rod with notch in tip to hold coil

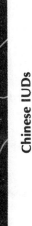

smallest A, to the largest D, and they have served as a standard for evaluating other IUDs.

HOW THE IUD WORKS

Until recently, the precise mechanisms by which IUDs prevented pregnancy remained unknown. This is partly because in animal studies the way the IUDs prevented pregnancy varied from species to species. In sheep and chickens they blocked sperm transport; in the guinea pig, cow, and pig they inhibited implantation; while in the guinea pig, rabbit, cow, and ewe they interfered with the function of the corpus luteum (the yellow egg sac in the ovary which secretes progesterone). Obviously several things were happening at the same time in some of these experiments. Recent research on humans has demonstrated that IUDs also affect ova and sperm in a variety of ways. They stimulate a foreign body inflammatory reaction in the uterus, not unlike the reaction experienced with a splinter in the finger. The concentration of white blood cells, prostaglandins, and enzymes that collect in response to the foreign body then interferes with the transport of sperm through the uterus and fallopian tubes and damages the sperm and ova, thus making fertilization impossible.[5]

CHANGES IN IUDS

In the 1970s a second generation of IUDs developed as the shift was made from the unmedicated Lippes Loop to copper-releasing IUDs and, to a lesser extent, to IUDs that release progestins into the uterine cavity. The copper devices had some advantages over the Lippes Loop since some of the copper IUDs are less likely to be expelled, produce less menstrual blood loss, are better tolerated by women who have not yet delivered babies, and are more likely to stay in place after postpartum or post-abortion insertion. The second generation of copper devices seemed to be slightly more effective than the Lippes Loop, though they still needed to be replaced more often and at a higher cost.

The new IUDs include those which release a steroid such as progesterone or synthetic hormones called progestins into the uterus.

THE CLINICAL INSERTION OF AN IUD

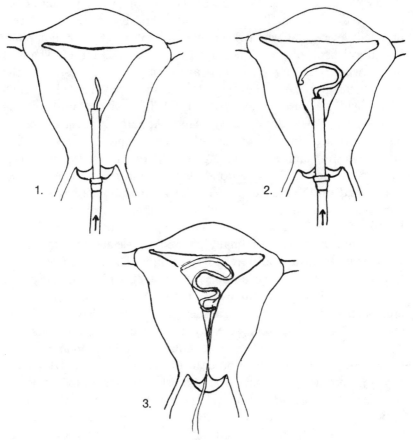

To position an IUD, the inserting device enters the cervical opening. The IUD is pushed into the uterus and expands to its full form.

Illustration by Steven Bullough

The effective doses of steroid are substantially lower than doses required for oral administration, and the systemic side effects are less frequent. The only hormone-releasing IUD currently marketed is Progestasert containing 38 mg. progestin released at a rate that calls for its replacement after one year. A long-lasting IUD using progestin is being widely tested but is not yet available for general use.

PROBLEMS

Problems arose in the 1970s over the use of IUDs, primarily because of the Dalkon Shield. This was a poorly designed, relatively untested device that was rushed onto the market by a major pharmaceutical firm, the A. H. Robins Company, to capture a share of the growing IUD market. Robins apparently did little testing of the product but purchased the rights to it from a physician, Dr. Hugh Davis, and his business associates in 1970, relying almost entirely on the testing allegedly done by Davis. Apparently most of the reports of testing were not particularly accurate and Davis was doing both the testing and the marketing, a violation of professional ethics. Though the device had questions raised about it almost as soon as it appeared on the market—insertion was exceptionally painful and there was a high rate of infection—complaints were initially ignored. By 1976, 17 deaths had been linked to its use, but Robins took no action until 1980 when it finally advised physicians to remove the shield from women who were still wearing it. The company's failure to act resulted in a large number of lawsuits, which ultimately led to Robins declaring bankruptcy.[6] In the aftermath of the Robins failure, other companies were also sued, and though lawsuits against other IUD manufacturers were not particularly successful, the liability insurance rates had risen so much that all companies in the United States ceased to distribute the devices for a time. IUDs were, however, available in Canada and in most of the rest of the world.

The major reason for the difference between the United States's response and that of the rest of the world is due largely to the fact that the United States is practically alone among the countries of the world in relying almost totally on private enterprise for its pharmaceuticals even though much of the research is paid for by the government. Obviously, private pharmaceutical companies want to sell IUDs for a profit. Since only a small percentage of American women used the device—approximately 7 percent in 1982–1983—and because IUDs are long-lasting, profits from any IUD after the initial adoption were modest. As more and more physicians switched to copper IUDs, sales of all plastic devices declined, leading the manufacturers of the Saf-T-Coil and the Lippes Loop to halt production for the American market. The Lippes Loop was particularly inexpensive and could be purchased in wholesale lots for less than a dollar a dozen. The Searle Company then took the copper Cu–7 and TCu–200 off the market temporarily because of lawsuits charging that the IUDs had injured their users.

One of the initial difficulties with IUDs was that no federal regulatory agency had any control over them. Drugs, including the pill, had to be approved by the Food and Drug Administration, which also supervised quality control of condoms. Since IUDs, however, were considered devices rather than drugs, FDA approval was not required prior to marketing them and the agency could only step in to ban such devices if they later proved hazardous to health. As a result IUDs could be promoted without adequate proof of safety and effectiveness. One result of the Dalkon Shield affair was the establishment of FDA rules to ensure that this could no longer happen. For example, the copper TCu–380A has been extensively tested and has proven to be one of the most effective methods of contraception ever developed. It was approved for sale by the Food and Drug Administration in 1984, although it took several years before a company, Gyno Pharma, Inc., was willing to market it in the United States. Rates of pregnancy were less than 1.0 per 100 women in the first year of use and, in the largest international study, only 1.4 after six years. The TCu–380A, along with others of the latest generation of IUDs—copper-bearing T-shaped devices including the TCu–220C, the Multiload–375, and the Nova T—are more effective in practice than oral contraceptives. This is also true of Progestasert. One advantage of Progestasert is that it increases serum iron levels. This might make it a desirable IUD for some women. Numerous other IUDs are being tested as of this writing.

SIDE EFFECTS

Early research indicated that IUD use increased the risk of Pelvic Inflammatory Disease (PID), an infection in the upper genital tract that can cause infertility. Recent studies have shown that the risk is largely limited to the first four months after IUD insertion and to those women who are exposed to a sexually transmitted disease. Women who fall into one of the following risk categories should not use the IUD: those who are pregnant or have had PID; those with a history of ectopic pregnancy, gynecological bleeding disorders, suspected malignancy of the genital tract, or congenital uterine abnormality; or women with fibroids that prevent proper IUD insertion. Other medical factors that might contra-indicate IUD use or require the judgment of both health care personnel and the potential users are: anemia (although here Progestasert would prove helpful), nulliparity (never having been pregnant), blood coagulation disorders, severe cervical stenosis, heavy menstrual flow, or severe primary dysmenorrhea. For those who are planning to use copper-bearing IUDs, copper allergy or Wilson's disease (a rare inherited disorder of copper excretion) are contra-indicators.[7] IUD users should be re-examined within three months after insertion and, after that, annual checks are useful. Women who have passed menopause should have their IUDs removed since narrowing and shrinking of the uterus may make later removal difficult and increase the chances of infection. The user should also periodically check for the IUD string and return for follow-up care if she cannot locate the string or if she misses a period.

EFFECTIVENESS

The IUD is, as indicated above, one of the most effective contraceptive methods. Though the device is relatively inexpensive, professional assistance is required to insert it, and the IUD should be checked periodically. For the individual woman, an IUD may be obtained free of charge through a family planning program or may cost as much as $100 from a private physician. The fact that IUDs are so inexpensive is just what makes them so favored among Third World countries, where their safety and effectiveness have long been demonstrated. American drug companies, however, are charging higher prices to cover their liability insurance costs.

CONCLUSION

An IUD is a good choice for the multiparous woman (one who has been pregnant and delivered at least once) who does not want to be bothered with daily procedures or pills. In some women who have never been pregnant it increases the menstrual flow and pain and irritates the cervix, thus making it a less desirable choice. The absence of the IUD from the American market for several years was due to panic on the part of the drug companies when the A. H. Robins Company was sued by so many people. As has been pointed out, Robins inadequately tested its product, and then was slow to listen to clients and physicians who complained. The other IUDs were never banned by the FDA, and current devices on the market are safe and effective. All such devices must now be approved by the FDA.

NOTES

1. Ernst Gräfenberg, "An Intrauterine Contraceptive Method," in M. Sanger and H. M. Stone, eds., *The Practice of Contraception: An International Symposium and Survey.* Proceedings of the Seventh International Birth Control Conference, Zurich, Switzerland, September 1930 (Baltimore, Md.: Williams and Wilkins, 1931), pp. 33–47.

2. T. Ota, "A Study on Birth Control with an Intrauterine Instrument," *Japanese Journal of Obstetrics and Gynecology* 17 (1934): 210–14.

3. Christopher Tietz and S. Lewit, eds., *Intra-uterine Contraceptive Devices.* Proceedings of the Conference, New York, April 30–May 1, 1962 (Amsterdam: Excerpta Medica, International Congress Series 54 [1962]).

4. Jack Lippes, "PID and the IUD." Paper presented at the World Congress of Gynecology and Obstetrics, Tokyo, October 1979.

5. World Health Organization (WHO), *Mechanization of Action, Safety and Efficacy of Intrauterine Devices* (Geneva: World Health Organization, 1987 [Technical Report Series 753]).

6. Morton Mintz, *At Any Cost: Corporate Greed, Women, and the Dalkon Shield* (New York: Pantheon Books, 1985).

7. International Planned Parenthood Federation (IPPF), International Medical Advisory Panel, "Statement on Intrauterine Devices," *IPPF Medical Bulletin* 16 (December 1981): 1–3.

6

Spermicides

Spermicides, as indicated in the opening chapter, are among the oldest and simplest of all techniques used to prevent conception. From ancient times to the present, various substances, usually highly acidic, with pastelike or sticky bases have been employed. The base plus an acid remain important elements in current spermicides. The historical efforts are particularly interesting because they started long before sperm were seen with the microscope and before the reproductive process was fully understood. The research was done on a trial and error basis, and the fact that ancient spermicides were developed attests to long-standing needs and desires for some kind of fertility control.

One of the first, if not the first, of the commercial spermicidal products were the quinine pessaries developed by English pharmacist Charles Rendell in 1885. These suppositories consisted of soluble cocoa butter plus quinine sulfate. Cocoa butter—a yellowish, hard, brittle vegetable fat obtained from the seeds of the *Theobroma cacao* plant—contains about 30 percent oleic acid, 40 percent stearic acid, as well as other fatty acids. It is a good vehicle for a spermicidal suppository because of its low melting point, and the cocoa butter itself probably served to block the cervix with an oily film. The quinine sulfate, however, was not a particularly potent spermicide and in some individuals it might have resulted in a toxic reaction. Other chemical combinations used as the active ingredient were chinosol, lactic acid, and boric acid.[1]

It was not until the 1920s that research into spermicides began seriously, and though the Rockefeller Foundation was one of the main

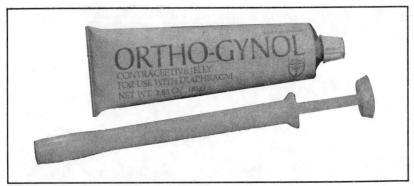

Example of one type of spermicidal jelly and its accompanying applicator.
Photograph courtesy of Ortho Pharmaceutical Corporation, Raritan, N.J.

supporters of such research it had to go to England and to Europe to find researchers willing to conduct tests, since the stigma attached to scientists in America who engaged in contraceptive research was so great.[2] European pharmaceutical firms also did research on their own.

Several refinements made spermicides somewhat more effective. The first was the development by a German pharmaceutical firm of a spermicide in combination with an effervescent tablet that foamed when it came in contact with moisture. The foam allowed widespread dispersal of the contraceptive in the vagina. In 1937, phenylmercuric acetate, a far more effective spermicide than quinine sulfate, was first used in the production of Volpar. Though this compound has since been banned from the U.S. market because of concerns about the safety of mercury, it proved very effective.[3]

A major breakthrough came with the introduction of surfacants, surface active agents, in the 1950s. These agents act primarily by disrupting the integrity of the sperm membrane. Since they are not strongly acidic they are rarely irritating to the vagina or penis, and they have become the principal active ingredient in spermicidal products. They can also be combined with different bases to make a wide variety of spermicides including jellies, suppositories, foaming tablets, and foams in pressurized containers.

Different types of spermicides vary in their ability to provide rapid and extensive coverage. Foams and jellies are dispersed best. Suppositories need body heat to melt. Foaming tablets need moisture to produce the foam, and distribution in the vagina may depend in part on coital movements. Thus, solid preparations may require as long as fifteen minutes between insertion and coitus to insure melting or foaming action. Dispersal, however, is also dependent on the amounts of vaginal fluids, and this varies from woman to woman.

ADVANTAGES

Spermicides can be purchased in the drugstore (as can condoms and sponges) without a prescription. Though prices vary, they are relatively inexpensive, costing approximately 50 cents to a dollar per use. They are not difficult to use and completely safe. These qualities are particularly important to first-time users. When combined with other easily available contraceptives, such as condoms, they are even more effective than when used alone. Many jellies, in fact, are designed to be used with barrier contraceptives.

TYPES OF SPERMICIDES

Foams

Contraceptive foams contain a spermicide that is injected into the vagina prior to coitus. A can of contraceptive foam should be shaken (directions usually call for shaking it twenty times) and then sprayed into an applicator and inserted well up into the vagina (close to the cervix). The foam must be injected into the vagina before intercourse and must remain there for six to eight hours after ejaculation. More foam should be inserted after each succeeding ejaculation.

Suppositories or Tablets

Contraceptive suppositories or tablets have to be inserted earlier in the lovemaking process than foam—at least ten minutes and not earlier than two hours before sex takes place. After insertion the suppository melts and fills the vagina with foam. A new suppository should be inserted for each act of intercourse. Women should avoid douching or bathing for several hours after ejaculation has taken place.

HOW TO INSERT SPERMICIDES

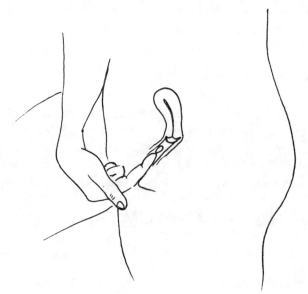

1. Inserting Suppository

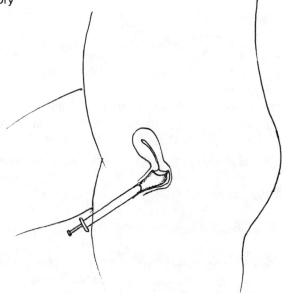

2. Inserting Jelly or Foam

Illustration by Steven Bullough

EFFECTIVENESS

Laboratory tests show that most spermicides do immobilize sperm, but clinical studies and use surveys yield failure rates from as low as 0.3 pregnancies per 100 woman-years of use to as high as nearly 40, depending on the products used, the populations tested, and the type of instruction and support that is provided. Obviously, the more closely the woman follows instructions and makes sure that the proper time elapses, the more effective the spermicides are. Most spermicidal contraceptives have as an active ingredient nonoxynol-9 or similar compounds that actually kill the sperm and, when used correctly, are very effective. Still, according to best estimates, the failure rate in the typical user is estimated at 15 per 100 woman-years, that is, 15 failures among 100 women using such a contraceptive over a year-long period. This rate obviously includes errors in use. Some misuses could be overcome with experience since reported failures have been due to such things as not removing the wrapping from suppositories or tablets, inserting the spermicide into the rectum instead of the vagina (perhaps because the term "suppository" is popularly associated with the rectum), not inserting the spermicide high enough into the vagina, having intercourse before the spermicide in suppositories or tablets is dispersed, having intercourse too long after insertion (when the product loses its effectiveness), not applying the spermicide before additional acts of intercourse, and not applying it during the supposedly infertile days of the menstrual cycle. Obviously, it is recommended that the would-be user carefully read the directions and even practice the using the spermicidal product before intercourse is contemplated.

Even with this failure rate, however, spermicides are more effective than *coitus interruptus,* fertility awareness techniques, douches, or simple chance where no method of fertility control is used. In the case of chance, the failure rate is 90 per 100 woman-years.

Occasionally one of the partners will be sensitive or allergic to the spermicidal jelly. A change of brand may help, but the formulas of the popular jellies are so similar that this does not ordinarily solve the problem. Couples who enjoy oral-genital sex may find the taste of spermicide unpleasant, although it is not harmful in small amounts. The other issue that has been raised in the literature is the possible link between spermicide use and congenital malformations of infants conceived in spite of the use of the spermicide, or fetuses who are exposed to the spermicides at a later date during the pregnancy. There are both positive and negative studies, with the current consensus being that there are no more abnormalties among the infants born of mothers who use the spermicides than are found in the general public. However, until more time has passed and more studies are done, it is prudent to avoid the spermicides if a pregnancy is known or suspected.[4]

Spermicides are becoming more important because of the current concern about sexually transmitted diseases. They are not totally effective in this regard but they very often protect against gonorrhea, syphilis, chlamydia, herpes, hepatitis B, and even AIDS.[5] Because of this protection, women who use a contraceptive jelly are less likely to develop pelvic inflammatory disease than are other women. The spermicides are even more effective as a prophylaxis against disease when they are combined with a barrier contraceptive.

SPERMICIDAL JELLY WITH A CONDOM, DIAPHRAGM, OR CERVICAL CAP

Contraceptive jelly (or gels) are most effective when combined with a barrier contraceptive such as a diaphragm, a cervical cap, or a condom. Only a small amount of gel is used with the cervical cap—a half teaspoon or less; the gel is put in the cap so it fills the inside area that touches the cervix. Similarly with the diaphragm, although a little bit of jelly around the edge of the diaphragm is important in establishing a barrier to sperm seeking to move around the rubber or plastic barrier. As indicated, most brands of spermicidal jelly include nonoxynol-9, which is both contraceptive and bacteriostatic. The use of a diaphragm or cervical cap, plus contraceptive gel, has a failure rate of less than 10 per one 100 woman-years. As noted above, the contraceptive gel also serves as a deterrent, but not absolute protection, against most sexually transmitted diseases.

If condoms are the barrier method of choice, the spermicide can be used in two different ways. There are now condoms that come with a small amount of spermicidal jelly as a lubricant. Since some kind of lubricant is needed to help the user slip the condom over the penis easily, a contraceptive gel is a good choice. The amount

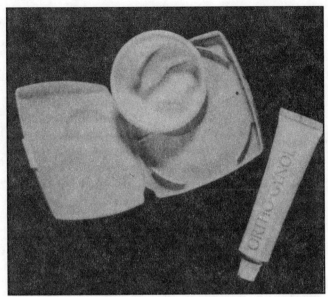

Diaphragm and Spermicide

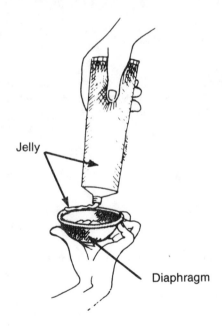

Jelly

Diaphragm

From Our Bodies, Ourselves, 1979. *Photograph and illustration reprinted by permission of the Boston Women's Health Book Collective.*

of contraceptive gel that can be used inside a condom, however, is so small that it offers only slightly better protection than the condom alone. A safer approach is to use a vaginal spermicide in the form of a suppository or foam along with the condom. Of course, to be very prudent, it is possible to use the spermicidal jelly as a lubricant and insert a vaginal spermicide also.

Most companies that manufacture vaginal gel also market a vaginal cream. While some women prefer the consistency of the cream, it is not advised for use with any barrier contraceptive, because creams are oil-based and thus destroy the rubber used in most barrier contraceptives.[6] Since the vaginal foams or suppositories are the safest of the spermicides if used without a barrier contraceptive, and the gels are better with diaphragms, caps, and condoms, the contraceptive creams are limited in their usefulness. Potential users could include those who employ oral contraceptives; sterile couples who use creams for their bacteriostatic and lubricant properties; and women who have just started oral contraceptives and need a back-up contraceptive for the first month, or during the first four months of IUD use.

NOTES

1. For a discussion of the early spermicides see Cecil I. B. Voge, *The Chemistry and Physics of Contraceptives* (London: Jonathan Cape, 1933).

2. See Vern L. Bullough, "Rockefellers and Sex Research," *Journal of Sex Research* 21 (May 1985): 113–25.

3. See "Spermicides—Simplicity and Safety Are Major Assets," *Population Reports,* Series H. Number 5 (September 1979): Volume 7, Number 5.

4. R. A. Hatcher, F. Guest, F. Stewart, G. K. Stewart, J. Trussell, S. C. Bowen, and W. Cates, *Contraceptive Technology 1988–1989* (New York: Irvington Publishers, 1988), pp. 323–31.

5. "Can You Rely on Condoms? *Consumer Reports* 54 (March 1989): 136–41.

6. B. Voeller, "Mineral Oil Lubricants Cause Rapid Deterioration of Latex Condoms," *Contraception* 39 (January 1989): 95–102.

7

Abstinence, Rhythm, and Natural Family Planning

The only abolutely sure-fire way to avoid pregnancy is abstinence, which in this sense means abstaining from heterosexual intercourse, not necessarily from all sex. Few people live lives of total abstinence, although Kinsey and his associates found that 2 percent of the women in his sample had never recognized any kind of sexual arousal under any condition and in the majority of cases had never had any contacts that could be identified as sexual. The researchers also found that 39 percent of the unmarried females over the age of forty-six had never experienced an orgasm at any time in their lives.[1]

Failure to have an orgasm, however, does not mean that the women abstained from sex entirely, since Kinsey also found that many married women with children reported not having an orgasm, although most of the 39 percent of unmarried females over forty-six in his sample probably had not engaged in sexual intercourse.

For single men the rates are not reported by Kinsey, except for certain age groups. He did find that one-third of the single men between thirty-one and thirty-five years of age were not engaging in sexual intercourse; this generalization would have held true for those who were older than thirty-five and unmarried.[2]

Some people who abstain from sexual intercourse do so for religious reasons: e.g., Catholic priests, monks, and nuns pledge themselves to a life of celibacy. Other individuals have low sexual drives, poor health, or find themselves in places (such as prisons and hospitals) where they cannot have heterosexual sex easily, or they have physical or mental conditions that make sex difficult. Even when all of these groups are included, lifelong abstinence from any kind of sexual activity is extremely rare. Many individuals who do not engage in heterosexual intercourse might engage in homosexual activities, masturbation, or petting to orgasm. Most men who consciously avoid all sexual activities have involuntary nocturnal emissions, or wet dreams.

Though few people adhere to a life of abstinence from all kinds of sexual activities, most have periods of greater or lesser abstinence during the childbearing ages. Young people, for example, are encouraged by society to abstain from intercourse until "they are mature enough to handle it" or, in many groups, until they are married. Homosexual men and lesbians are encouraged to be abstinent by those who disapprove of such sexual activity. Older people who have lost their sexual partners or who live in homes for senior citizens are often expected to be abstinent, as are married people who are separated from each other because of employment or illness or other factors. The list could go on although obviously what society says about the importance of abstinence and what people do are quite often different. When we talk about abstinence in terms of contraception, however, we mean planned periodic abstention from sexual intercourse.

For some highly motivated couples, periodic abstinence is the preferred method of family planning. For others abstinence within a relationship is not acceptable even though they might have theoretically agreed to adopt the method. This results in a high proportion of failures. The term "failure," however, might be misleading since those involved in natural family planning, as advocates of periodic abstinence call their methods, label such failures as "informed choice pregnancies." This is because the couple involved in natural family planning knows the rules for avoiding pregnancy, and if they avoid following the rules, then they simply are "asking for a child."

Natural family planning relies upon periodic abstinence and requires two things for success: (1) identifying the fertile period occurring at the time of the ovulation, usually about fourteen days before the onset of the next menstrual period, and (2) abstaining from sexual intercourse for several days before and after the expected date of ovulation.

Technically, it was not until the 1930s, when Kyusaku Ogino in Japan and Hermann Knaus in Austria independently identified the time of ovulation in relation to the menstrual cycle, that any kind of periodic abstinence held a better chance for controlling births than pure chance.[3] Since the period of fertility coincides in general with ovulation, it should be simple to plot the cycle on the calendar and have intercourse only during the nonfertile phases. Unfortunately, it is based upon estimating when ovulation will occur or has occurred, and this date can only be definitively known when the next menstrual period begins, which is some 14 days after ovulation. Some women have regular periods at 28- or 29-day intervals, while others experience much more variation. Since this is the case, there are long periods in the cycle requiring abstinence; much effort has been expended in trying to calculate more accurately when ovulation will or has occurred to cut down on abstinence. Because the rhythm method does not interfere with the natural cycle in any way and is a way of choosing rather than controlling conception, it is the only method approved by the Roman Catholic Church. The methods developed to help predict ovulation, in fact, are very helpful to those people who are trying to get pregnant. There are various ways of attempting to predict when ovulation is likely to occur, and most individuals who adopt the rhythm method use a combination of these predictive approaches.

CALENDAR RHYTHM

Most advocates of the calendar rhythm method follow the formula developed by the Japanese researcher Ogino rather than that advocated by Knaus, since Ogino stipulated additional days of abstinence in order to allow for a longer possible fertile period resulting from the variation in time of ovulation. According to Ogino's formula, a woman estimates the beginning of her fertile period by subtracting eighteen days from the shortest previous six to twelve menstrual cycles, and the end of the fertile period by subtracting eleven days from the longest cycle. This does not mean that she is actually fertile all of those days but that the fertile period will fall into that time span.

Example 1

The average length of menstrual cycle for subject X over the past 12 months is 23 to 31 days.

$$31 - 11 = 20 \qquad\qquad 23 - 18 = 5$$

This means that X's fertile period could take place any time from 5 days after the beginning of her menses until 20 days after. The couple should not engage in intercourse from the fifth day after the beginning of the menses until the 21st day, for a total abstention of 16 days.

Example 2

Subject Y has a more regular menstrual cycle with a range between 27 and 29 days over the past 12 months.

$$29 - 11 = 18 \qquad\qquad 27 - 18 = 9$$

This couple would abstain beginning 9 days after the onset of the menses and could begin again on the 19th day, thus they would have only a 10-day period of abstinence. This is the minimum amount of abstinence possible under the calendar system.

Problems with the Calendar Rhythm Method

If the menses are always regular, the system might be foolproof for those who practice it, but the difficulty is that many women have cycles like the one given in the first example. Unfortunately also, all sorts of factors can influence the menses of women who usually are quite regular: tension, illness, anxiety, stress, and the like. This makes the method less successful than it should be in theory. The calendar method also requires a dedication by both partners to observe the rules of the game, but not all do. As a result, the failure rate is among the highest of any method of contraception. Almost 18.8 percent, or nearly one in five women, become pregnant within the first year of using the calendar method. Still, this is a lower rate than would have occurred without using the method, since it is estimated that anywhere from 50 to 85 percent of sexually active women would become pregnant within a year if no method at all were used.[4]

Usually the calendar method is supplemented by other methods aimed at predicting when ovulation will occur more accurately in order to cut down on the days that abstinence is required and to take into account the occasional irregularities in the menstrual cycle.

THE TEMPERATURE METHOD

This method is based on an observation first made in 1868 that women's basal body temperature (BBT), that is, the temperature of the body at rest, rises slightly during the later part of the menstrual cycle.[5] It was not until the 1930s, however, that this rise in temperature was linked to ovulation, whereupon daily recording of temperatures were suggested to users of the calendar rhythm method as a way of better identifying the fertile period.[6] The woman using the BBT method charts her daily temperature and abstains from intercourse between the first day of menstruation and the third consecutive day of elevated temperatures. Her temperature begins to rise one to two days after ovulation in response to rising levels of the hormone progesterone. Though there might be some safe days during and immediately after the menses, under this system intercourse is not advised from the onset of menstruation because the BBT does not predict when ovulation would occur but only when it has happened, and it is easier to date the beginning of the menses than its end. The three-day wait after the temperature rise is intended to assure that the ovum is no longer fertilizable. Used by itself the method allows for about ten safe days of intercourse every cycle before the menses begin again. When combined with the calendar method, however, it has the advantage of allowing an earlier resumption of sexual activity and would also permit intercourse during and immediately following the menses, allowing for fewer days of abstinence. There are, however, advocates of the temperature method who prefer to rely upon it and not combine it with the calendar method. This means that there are about eighteen days of abstinence during each cycle.[7]

Problems with the Temperature Method

Success with the temperature method depends upon (1) how carefully daily temperatures are taken and recorded, and (2) how well a woman can recognize the rise in BBT. This takes some skill and training, since the temperature rise is slight (from two tenths to four tenths of a degree Centigrade or from four tenths to eight tenths of a degree Fahrenheit). (3) Success is also determined by how closely the rise in temperature concides with ovulation. The calculation of change in temperature has been made much easier by the development of special thermometers with expanded scales that allow slight changes to be more easily detected. Though the BBT can be taken orally, rectally, or vaginally, the rectal temperature is the most accurate. It should, however, be taken at roughly the same time every morning after at least three to five hours of uninterrupted sleep. Any deviations from the routine or from a regular pattern of behavior can affect the BBT, and such factors should be noted on the daily chart. Anything from a mild illness to extreme changes in environmental temperature to unexplained modifications in the body's regulating system can affect the BBT. Still, for women who are faithful in recording their daily temperature and whose partners are willing to abstain from sex during more than half the menstrual cycle, the BBT method by itself is far more effective than the calendar method. It is the long period of abstinence from sexual intercourse that actually creates the greatest problem. For this reason, few couples rely upon the temperature method alone but prefer to combine it with the calendar method, which allows for more safe days. The temperature method, however, is particularly valuable in planning pregnancies since it pinpoints the most fertile period.

THE CERVICAL MUCUS METHOD

Just as there are changes in basal body temperature, changes take place in the cervical mucus in response to the changing hormonal levels. Two Australian physicians, John and Evelyn Billings, developed a method of periodic abstinence based solely on the cervical mucus changes.[8] In a typical menstrual cycle, the secretory cells in the cervix produce two kinds of mucus at two different phases, and each type has its own cellular and chemical components as well as physical structure. During most of the cycle the mucus is designed to act as a barrier to the entrance of sperm, but following ovulation the purpose is to encourage entrance of sperm.

Once menstrual bleeding has stopped, there is little or no mucus for a few days. Then a white or cloudy and tacky mucus is discharged; the amount increases over the next few days. The mucus then becomes thinner and clearer and it increases in amount. There are one or two days when the mucus is thin like raw egg white, slippery and elastic. Because of its stretchability it has been termed *spinnbarkheit* mucus. It somewhat resembles the fluid produced during sexual arousal. Ovulation occurs at the end of this clear mucus period. After ovulation the mucus thickens, becoming cloudy and white. It also loses its elasticity.

Changes in mucus are due to changing hormone levels. During the preovulatory and ovulatory phases, the mucus is Type E or estrogenic. It is responding to ovarian secretions of estrogen. After ovulation, when progesterone is produced, the mucus is known as Type B or gestagenic, and this marks the beginning of the safe period. A woman using this method has to learn to distinguish between two types of mucus, both by feeling inside her vagina as well as by visual inspection. To confirm her feeling sensations, she should remove ex-cretions from her vagina with a tissue or her finger in order to check its appearance and stretchiness. Learning to recognize mucus patterns takes some time (often several months of instruction and practice) and abstinence is recommended during the entire first month of instruction. To be effective, abstinence should begin on the first day after menses that mucus is observed (wet mucus, Type E, appears first) and continue until three days after the *spinnbarkheit* type of mucus disappears.

Problems with the Cervical Mucus Method

The method by itself takes a long time to learn and until the woman is comfortable with it, mistakes are likely to be made. Even the most dedicated follower, however, runs up against the problem of variations in the body's response patterns. Since sperm may survive in the reproductive tract up to three days (and perhaps longer), the advent of the *spinnbarkheit* may come too late to warn the couple that attempts coitus during the first part of the cycle. Another reason for failure is a misinterpretation of the mucus since patterns of mucus can be affected by a variety of physiological and psychological factors. Again, however, the method is particularly valuable for planning

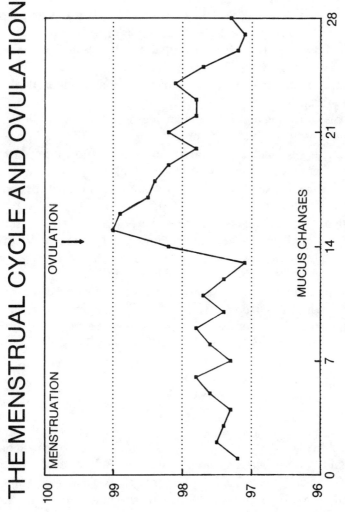

THE MENSTRUAL CYCLE AND OVULATION

Ovulation occurs about 14 days before the beginning of the next menstrual period.
Chart shows a 28-day cycle

pregnancies when intercourse should coincide and immediately follow ovulation as indicated by the *spinnbarkheit*.

THE SYMPTO-THERMAL METHOD

For those following natural family planning methods, the sympto-
thermal method or STM is the best since it combines all the previously
mentioned methods into one. It uses the calendar calculations and
supplements them by using the thermal (temperature) and mucus
changes. This allows many women reasonably to predict the day
ovulation will take place and to double-and triple-check their
observations. Available STM charts allow a person to record the
changes in basal body temperature, cervical mucus, mid-cycle spotting
and pain, changes in the cervix, and menstruation and intercourse.
Different organizations have developed their own instructions and
charts. The one developed by the World Health Organization calls
for abstinence beginning with the calendar calculations or when the
thin mucus is first noted, whichever comes earlier. The calendar
calculations are figured in the manner indicated above, and intercourse can resume after ovulation in accordance with both the temperature and mucus methods. This is calculated by using either the
fourth day after the peak mucus symptom or the evening of the third
day of consecutive high temperatures (which are taken in the morning), whichever is later.

Problems with the Sympto-Thermal Method

STM is difficult to learn because it combines so many different
monitoring systems and sometimes gives contradictory information.
It takes a considerable period of guidance and supervision before
most women can use it. Long periods of abstinence are also required.
Still, the STM method is the most effective natural family planning
method, and if it is combined with calendar calculations, abstinence
is unnecessary during menstruation, thus giving a greater number
of days in which safe intercourse can take place.

OTHER INDICATORS

In addition to the body changes taking place in the methods discussed above, there are indicators mentioned in the chapter on anatomy and physiology that are useful to some women who follow natural family planning methods. Some women can tell when they ovulate through the appearance of an abdominal pain known technically as *mittelschmerz* or "middle pain." For those women who have such pain regularly, the ability to sense it can be accentuated through careful instruction and it becomes a useful supplement to accuracy.

A few women also have menstrual spotting shortly before, during, or right after ovulation; this can be used to focus in on the fertile period. Such bleeding, however, is not always consistent during the cycle and can occur for other reasons. There are also cyclical changes in the cervix, which can be observed with the help of a speculum and mirror: they include softening, dilation, shift in position, and wetness, all of which signify ovulation.

A NEW METHOD

More hopeful has been the recent development of self-administered tests to detect hormonal changes. Enzyme immunoassays for urinary estrogen and pregnanediol glucoronide have recently been developed that can be easily used at home at minimal cost and require minimal time to perform. Such tests have to be performed by the woman about twelve days each month, but they should reduce the number of days of abstinence required.[9] It is not yet clear to what extent this aid to natural planning will be used when it becomes generally available. Since it involves purchasing of various kits, widespread use is possible since the pharmaceutical companies, who so far have not found much profit in the natural family planning methods, will push it. It will also be much easier to perform than the cervical mucus observations.

Combining the various techniques described above in order to identify fertility periods with either the use of barrier contraceptives or *coitus interruptus* during the fertile phase should lessen the period of abstinence. However, using a barrier contraceptive would not be accepted by many of the groups advising natural family planning methods.

NATURAL FAMILY PLANNING METHODS: A SUMMATION

There are both advantages and disadvantages to using natural family planning methods. The advantages would include the fact that there are no physical side effects for the users, costs are minimal, and training in the methods increases awareness and knowledge of reproductive functions. Since they involve close collaboration between husband and wife, these methods might also emphasize the need for a mutual partnership in marriage. For some people the methods may seem more esthetically acceptable and, perhaps most important of all, they are morally acceptable to the Roman Catholic Church and therefore to couples who want to adhere to the church's teaching.

With respect to their disadvantages, the natural family planning methods are simply not as effective as other contraceptive methods in avoiding pregnancy. They require long periods of training and orientation, necessitate daily monitoring and long-term commitment to the project, demand cooperation of both partners, and require sexual abstinence that can cause psychological stress and marital difficulty. It should be added that women with irregular menstrual cycles will have difficulty in using the methods. Those women who are fairly regular, and whose partners support these methods, will have the most success.

Another problem with natural family planning is that there is still some uncertainty about how long sperm that are lodged in the female genital tract remain viable and capable of union with an ovum. The current belief is that sperm maintain their ability to fertilize for approximately forty-eight hours, but it may be possible under certain favorable conditions for sperm to retain their power to fertilize for as long as five days and perhaps even longer. If sperm remain capable of fertilizing ova for more than three days, women using any of the natural family planning methods are at greater risk of pregnancy than the current techniques assume. Future research will, we hope, solve this problem by furnishing more accurate data.

The other problem that research could help solve is the uncertainty involved in predicting ovulation. If it could be predicted three days ahead of time and if the sperm were known with certainty to be viable for only forty-eight hours, the period of abstinence could be cut to less than five days.

Since training in these methods is essential, readers interested in in them or in finding help should contact the Natural Family Planning Center of Washington, D.C. (8514 Bradmoor Drive, Bethesda, Maryland 20817), the Pope Paul VI Institute for Study of Human Reproduction (6901 Mercy Road, Omaha, Nebraska 68106), Northwest Natural Family Planning Service, Inc. (4805 Blisan Street, N.E., Portland, Oregon 97213 [Sympto-Thermal Method]), or the International Family of the Americas Foundation (1150 Lover's Lane, P.O. Box 219, Mandeville, Louisiana 70448 [Billings Method]). Most Catholic Family Service Agencies also have information available.

NOTES

1. A. C. Kinsey, W. B. Pomeroy, C. E. Martin, and P. H. Gebhard, *Sexual Behavior in the Human Female* (Philadelphia: W. B. Saunders, 1953), pp. 512–13, 526.

2. A. C. Kinsey, W. B. Pomeroy, and C. E. Martin, *Sexual Behavior in the Human Male* (Philadelphia: W. B. Saunders, 1948), pp. 706–709.

3. K. Ogino, "Ovulationstermin und Konzeptionstermin," *Zentralbaltt für Gynäkologie* 54 (February 1930): 464–79; H. Knaus, "Die periodische Frucht-und Unfruchtbarkeit des Weibes," *Zentralbaltt für Gynäkologie* 54 (June 1933): 1393.

4. W. R. Grady, M. B. Hirsch, N. Keen, and B. Vaughan, "Differentials in Contraceptive Use Failure among Married Women Aged 15–44 Years; United States, 1970–76," Washington, D.C.: National Center for Health Statistics, 1981, and cited in "Periodic Abstinence," *Population Reports,* Series 1, Number 3 (September 1981): Volume 9, Number 4.

5. W. Squire, "Puerperal Temperatures," *Transactions of the Obstetrical Society (London)* 9 (1868): 129.

6. J. Ferin, "Détermination de la période stérile prémenstruelle par la courbe thermique," *Bruxelles Medica* 27 (1947): 86–93.

7. "Periodic Abstinence," *Population Reports* 9 (1981): 4, Series 1, Number 3.

8. J. Billings, *Natural Family Planning: The Ovulation Method* (Collegeville, Minn.: Liturgical Press, 1973). This is a thirty-eight-page pamphlet. See also a book (96 pages) by Billings, *The Ovulation Method* (Melbourne, Australia: Advocate Press, 1979), and E. Billings and A. Westmore, *The Billings Method: Controlling Fertility without Drugs or Devices* (New York: Random House, 1980).

9. J. B. Brown, L. F. Blackwell, J. J. Billings, et al., "Natural Family Planning," *American Journal of Obstetrics and Gynecology* 157 (1987): 1082–89.

8

The Condom

The condom has been around for a long time, as was indicated in chapter 1. The modern condom did not exist until methods for making rubber latex were developed in the middle of the nineteenth century. Since the rubber condom was regarded as a sexual device—unlike the diaphragm, which could be patented as a pessary—it was an under-the-counter invention. Its history can only be traced through literary references, and though it was possible to make a latex condom in 1853, the first reference to such a device was in 1858.[1] This original latex condom was an "apex" envelope and was described as being made of a "delicate texture" rubber no thicker than the cuticle, shaped and bounded at the open end with an Indian rubber ring and designed to fit over the tip of the penis. The cap was soon extended to cover the shaft of the penis as does the modern condom. One of the earliest, if not the earliest, mention of a full-length rubber condom is in 1869. These early condoms were molded from sheet crepe and carried a seam along their entire length.

Making the rubber condom more effective and useful depended on further developments in rubber technology, particularly the seamless cement process, so named because the process was similar to that used in producing rubber cement. In this process natural rubber was ground up, dissolved, then heated with solvent into which cylindrical glass molds were dipped. As the solvents evaporated, the condoms dried. They were then vulcanized by being exposed to sulfur dioxide (which added to the rubber's strength and elasticity). A similar process was used in making rubber surgical gloves, which appeared

107

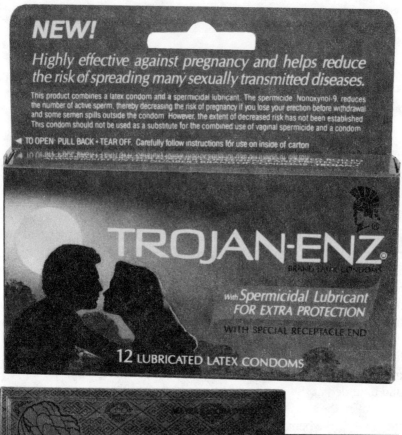

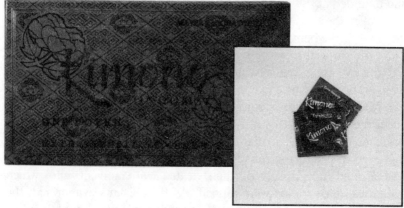

The condoms shown represent two of many varieties and brands currently on the market. They are individually wrapped, can be purchased over the counter in varying quantities, and include instructions on proper use.

The photographs are reproduced courtesy of Carter-Wallace, Inc., New York, N.Y. (Trojan) and Mayer Laboratories, Oakland, Calif. (Kimono).

on the market in 1889.[2] Seamless condoms probably preceded the manufacture of rubber gloves although the sources are silent about these underground innovations. The process of dipping was time-consuming as well as hazardous to workers since the solvents were highly flammable. The major defect of the finished product was that it deteriorated rather rapidly. Still the condoms were relatively inexpensive and disposable, and the seamless rubber method remained the standard manufacturing technique until well into the twentieth century. Fortunately, some of the dangers to workers were lessened by further mechanization of the process.

In the United States the early condoms were primarily peddled as prophylactics, that is, as disease preventatives, rather than contraceptives, although early descriptions recognize this function as well. As prophylactics, condoms were available in brothels as well as in drugstores, where they went by such euphemisms as French letters or capotes. They were also often sold in barber shops and other places where only men ventured. The problem with the early condoms was quality control since there was neither copyright nor patent protection. None of the major manufacturers of rubber in the United States, at least as indicated by the materials in their archives available at the University of Akron,[3] manufactured condoms, and this meant that the market was left to a number of smaller companies, some of which had very tenuous financial bases. Eventually several companies emerged with adequate quality control, including Young's Rubber, Julius Schmid, and Akwell. The entrance of Young's Rubber, founded by Merle Young (a drugstore products salesman) in the mid-1920s, was particularly important since he was able to convince druggists to sell his condoms by promising effective quality control over his product. Young's Rubber also began a series of court suits that eventually overturned many of the laws against condom sales.

In the 1930s, new techniques were developed that enabled rubber plantations to ship concentrated liquid natural rubber latex directly to the manufacturer, and this eliminated the need to grind and dissolve rubber back to a liquid state. Though this proved to be a less costly method of manufacture, the problem of quality control remained. In one of the first American surveys of the efficacy of condoms, that of the National Committee on Maternal Health in 1938, it was found that only about 40 percent of the rubber condoms sold in the United

States were fit for use.[4] One result of such a finding was the decision to assign the U.S. Food and Drug Administration control over the quality of condoms sold or shipped in interstate commerce. Federal policy in effect turned full circle: After first trying to outlaw contraceptive information and, when this was no longer possible, ignoring the existence of such things as condoms, the government finally recognized that condoms were an important consumer product. The first government effort to look at quality control found that as much as 75 percent of the condoms then on the market had small pinholes caused either by the existence of dust particles in the liquid latex or by improperly vulcanized latex.[5] This situation changed rapidly.

By the 1960s, condoms were among the most effective contraceptives on the market. They were simple to use, easy to buy, inexpensive, and did not require a physical examination or a physician's advice. Since they simply served as a container for the semen and did not interfere with any of the bodily processes, they were also harmless. In spite of these assets, use of condoms declined in the 1960s and 1970s in the United States, as did barrier contraceptives in general, due for the most part to the emergence of oral contraceptives. New emphasis was given to the use of condoms in the 1980s with the appearance of Acquired Immune Deficiency Syndrome (AIDS) as well as new outbreaks of more traditional sexually transmitted diseases (herpes, gonorrhea, etc.). Because condoms not only prevent sperm from entering the vagina, but also prevent the passage of the HIV (AIDS) virus and other disease-causing organisms, public health professionals urge the use of a condom for all sexual encounters outside of long-standing monogamous relationships. This advice holds even if other contraceptives are also used, and applies to both heterosexual and homosexual activities including penile-anal sex, which has been involved in the spread of the HIV virus. The potential effectiveness of condoms in preventing the spread of sexually transmitted diseases led the U.S. government in the decade of the eighties to impose particularly stringent quality controls on the manufacturers of condoms in an effort to eliminate failure when a condom is used correctly.

Originally all condoms came in one size, and the assumption of one-size-fits-all was only challenged when the United States began exporting condoms to Asian countries and found that they were too large for many Asian men. In Thailand, for example, the oversized condoms became such a publicized joke that comedians reported that men had to use a "string to tie the condoms to their waist for the sake of safety."[6] Upon more scientific investigation it was found that the median erect penis length of Thai men was between 126 and 150 mm., while that of U.S. men was between 151 and 175 mm. The median erect penis circumference of Thai men was between 101 and 112 mm.; U.S. men measured between 113 and 137 mm. (25.40 mm. = 1 inch).[7] Most large international manufacturers now produce two basic sizes, Class I, 180 mm. in length and 52 mm. in flat width, and Class II, 160 mm. in length and 49 mm. in flat width. In the United States some manufacturers are offering the smaller-size condoms by promoting them as fitting "snugger for extra sensitivity" rather than indicating they are for men with smaller sized penises. Rubber membranes can be produced as thin as .03 mm. but most range from .04 to .07. They are produced in various styles: dry or lubricated, plain or reservoir-ended, straight or shaped, smooth or textured, colored or natural. Consumers Union, which rated condoms in their magazine *Consumer Reports* in March 1989, found that its readers preferred lubricated condoms with a reservoir tip, although a substantial minority liked extra-thin, extra-strong, or lubricated spermicidal condoms. These ratings appear on pages 112–113 of this book.

USE

Condoms, like any other barrier contraceptive, require some skill in use. First-time users should read the instructions in the condom package in the daylight and well before planning to use one. In fact, it is a good idea to practice putting one on before trying to use one the first time (the practice condom should then be discarded). Most condoms are prerolled. Those without the reservoir tip should be unrolled for about a half inch before placing it on the penis. This procedure allows for space at the end to collect the sperm. For a man who is not circumcised, the foreskin must be pulled back from the penis before putting the condom on. The condom should be placed over the erect penis and unrolled down the shaft. It should slide on easily and not get bound up. If it does, it is being put on the wrong way and another condom should be tried. Some couples find

GUIDE TO THE RATINGS

Grouped by projected failure rate in airburst testing, adjusted statistically for number of samples tested; within groups, listed in order of decreasing volume and pressure withstood in test. Differences between closely ranked models are not significant.

1 **Price.** Average price CU shoppers paid in New York City area stores for one dozen condoms.

2 **Lubrication.** Some models come with "dry" lubrication (**D**), typically a silicon-based oil. Others are wet-lubricated (**W**), with a water-based surgical jelly.

3 **Spermicide.** These models contain the spermicide nonoxynol-9, but concentrations and amounts vary. Most labels say that their spermicide lubricant is no substitute for the use of vaginal spermicide.

4 **Texture.** Ribbing or stippling around the shaft.

5 **Contour.** Shapes varied considerably. Some condoms are flared, others tapered, yet others have contouring for more snug fit.

6 **Variability.** Inconsistencies included: large differences in airburst performance among lots tested (**A**); color variations among or within packages (**C**); lubrication variations within packages (**L**); shape variations among or within packages (**S**); and texture variations among or within packages (**T**). Some models come in strips, and in some lots it was hard to separate the individual packets (**P**). For some models, we didn't test enough lots to check lot-to-lot differences in airburst results (**X**).

SPECIFICATIONS AND FEATURES

Except as noted, all: • Have reservoir tip. • Showed small lot-to-lot variation in strength. • Did not vary among or within packages in color, lubrication, or texture. • Had opaque individual packet. • Were sealed in individual packets, packed in strips, and easy to separate and open. • Had a slight odor. • Have a natural latex color.

KEY TO COMMENTS

A—Instructions judged better than most.
B—Instructions judged worse than most.
C—Packets translucent; could hasten aging.
D—Packets transparent; could hasten aging.
E—Individual packets not sealed; could hasten aging.
F—Many packets not airtight; could hasten aging.
G—Individual packets hard to open.
H—Has unpleasant odor.
I—Had thin spots.
J—Comes in assorted colors (**Excita Fiesta, Wrinkle Zero-0 2000, Yamabuki No. 2**); comes in pink (**Protex Arouse**); comes in golden yellow (**Trojans Plus, Trojan Ribbed**).
K—Comes with wallet for purse or pocket.
L—Has plain tip.
M—Thinner than most (roughly, 0.05 mm).
N—Thicker than most (roughly, 0.08 mm or more).
O—Has applicator and adhesive to hold condom on penis.

Reprints of this report will be available in bulk quantity. For information and prices, write CU/Reprints, P.O. Box CS 2010-A, Mount Vernon, N.Y. 10551.

RATINGS—Latex Condoms

Brand and model	Price (1)	Lubrication (2)	Spermicide (3)	Texture (4)	Contour (5)	Variability (6)	Comments
■ *The following models had a projected maximum failure rate of 1.5 percent.*							
Gold Circle Coin	$2.75	—	—	—	—	X	A,E,N
LifeStyles Extra Strength Lubricated	5.63	D	—	—	—	—	N
Saxon Wet Lubricated	4.47	W	—	—	—	X	B,G
Ramses Non-Lubricated Reservoir End	5.96	—	—	—	—	S,X	F
Sheik Non-Lubricated Reservoir End	3.43	—	—	—	—	P,X	F
Excita Extra	6.60	D	✔	✔	—	P	A,C
Kimono	7.64	D	—	—	✔	X	A,D,G
Sheik Elite	4.83	D	✔	—	—	—	A,C,M
Koromex with Nonoxynol-9	6.56	D	✔	—	—	—	C,K
Excita Fiesta	6.77	D	—	✔	—	P,X	C,J
Embrace Ultra-Thin	3.36	D	—	—	✔	L	B,C,F
LifeStyles Stimula Vibra-Ribbed	5.08	D	—	✔	—	P	B,C
Ramses Extra with Spermicidal Lubricant	5.80	D	✔	—	—	P	A,C
Lady Trojan	5.25	W	✔	—	—	X	A,F,H
Trojan Plus 2	5.25	W	✔	—	✔	X	A
Protex Secure	4.32	D	—	—	—	C,S	C,F,H
Protex Touch	3.87	D	—	—	—	—	C,H
Protex Arouse	4.00	D	—	✔	✔	C,S,T	C,J
Trojan-Enz	3.56	—	—	—	—	—	—
Lady Protex with Spermicidal Lubricant	4.14	D	✔	—	—	C	C,H
Sheik Fetherlite Snug-Fit	5.42	D	—	—	✔	P,X	C
Trojan Naturalube Ribbed	5.30	W	—	✔	✔	—	H
Protex Contracept Plus with Spermicidal Lubricant	4.61	D	✔	—	—	C	C,H
Lady Protex Ultra-Thin	3.97	D	—	—	—	C,X	C,H
Trojan-Enz Lubricated	4.41	W	—	—	—	—	H
Trojan Ribbed	5.15	D	—	✔	—	—	D,J
Today with Spermicidal Lubricant	6.16	D	✔	—	✔	X	A,G,I
LifeStyles Conture	4.28	D	—	—	✔	—	B,C
Trojans	3.74	—	—	—	—	—	L
Trojans Plus	5.07	D	—	—	✔	—	D,J
Yamabuki No. 2 Lubricated	7.32	D	—	—	✔	X	A,C,J,M
Wrinkle Zero-0 2000	7.32	D	—	✔	✔	—	A,C,J
■ *The following models had a projected maximum failure rate of 4 percent.*							
Sheik Non-Lubricated Plain End	4.08	—	—	—	—	—	L
Ramses Sensitol Lubricated	5.82	D	—	—	✔	P,S,X	C
Pleaser Ribbed Lubricated [1]	3.46	D	—	✔	✔	—	C,F
Ramses NuFORM	6.26	D	—	—	✔	P	C
Mentor	18.62	D	—	—	—	—	A,O
LifeStyles Nuda	4.69	D	—	—	✔	—	B,C
■ *The following models had a projected maximum failure rate of more than 10 percent.*							
LifeStyles Extra Strength with Nonoxynol-9	8.07	D	✔	—	—	A	F,I,N
LifeStyles Nuda Plus	5.40	D	✔	—	✔	A	A,C,I

[1] Now called **Saxon Ribbed Lubricated.**

HOW TO PUT ON A CONDOM

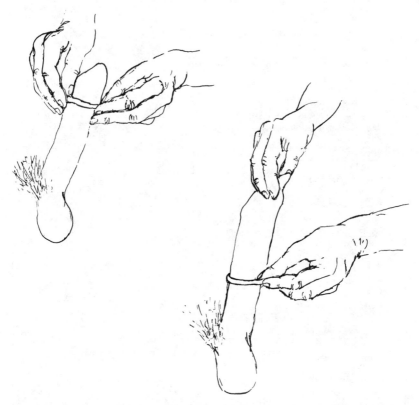

Fit the condom over the head of the penis after having reserved a small space at the tip to hold the ejaculate. Once positioned, the remainder of the condom is rolled down the shaft of the penis.

Illustration by Steven Bullough

it erotically stimulating for the partner to help put on the condom before intercourse takes place. This procedure also allows the condom to become part of the sexual foreplay instead of an interruption. After ejaculation, the man must withdraw from the vagina before the penis becomes flaccid or soft. While withdrawing, he should hold the condom firmly in place with his fingers at the base of the penis so that it will not slip off or leak sperm. After the condom is removed, the penis should not touch any part of the woman's vagina because the penis may have live sperm on it. Do not flush the condom down the toilet since it could clog the plumbing. Do not use the same condom twice. Some condoms come with a spermicide in their lubricant but it is no substitute for a vaginal spermicide, and the woman is advised to use an over-the-counter spermicide (such as nonoxynol–9) in addition to her partner's use of the condom.

When using a condom certain things should be avoided. For example, some people like to lubricate the condom with such materials as vaseline, but these weaken and dissolve the latex. If a lubricant is desired, make sure it is one that is water based, such as K-Y jelly, and not oil based like petroleum jelly. The same advice holds for spermicides as well. Any jelly or spermicide that can be safely used with a diaphragm, which is also made of latex, is suitable for the condom.

PROBLEMS

Decreased sensitivity is a common complaint of males and, to a lesser extent, of females in intercourse where the condom is used. For some men, however, decreased sensitivity is an advantage since it tends to prolong intercourse. Whether condoms do reduce sensation and by how much is something that has never been effectively measured. Users who are bothered by this might turn to the thinner condoms and to the prelubricated ones. Another objection is the inconvenience or troublesomeness of the method since many complain that it requires an interruption of lovemaking to put one on. As indicated above, this can be at least partially solved by including the condom as part of the erotic foreplay of lovemaking.

EFFECTIVENESS

For those who use condoms consistently the pregnancy rates are low, between 0.7 and 3.6 per 100 couple-years (the term used for male-oriented contraceptives). This means that between 0.7 and 3.6 of every hundred couples using the contraceptive will be involved in a pregnancy during any one year.[8] For those who use condoms only occasionally or inconsistently the pregnancy rates are much higher. The

National Survey of Family Growth found that 9.6 percent of condom users experienced an accidental pregnancy in the first year of use, and part of this failure was probably due to inexperience in their use.[9]

Effectiveness, as in so many other forms of contraception, depends upon knowledge and willingness to follow the procedures. Experience helps. Since there are so many condoms on the market, it might be that some users will find one brand or type more comfortable or erotic than others. Condoms are not particularly expensive, from $4 to $10 per dozen, although more expensive cecum condoms, made from animal intestinal tissue, are also available. They work as well as the latex ones in preventing pregnancy but not as well in preventing the transmission of disease (such as AIDS). A good survey of available brands was reported on in *Consumer Reports*.[10] The report included readers' preferences, which mght be helpful to new users of condoms.

NOTES

1. Vern L. Bullough, "A Brief Note on Rubber Technology and Contraception: The Diaphragm and the Condom," *Technology and Culture* 22 (January 1981): 104–111.

2. See Vern L. Bullough and Bonnie Bullough, "How Rough Red Hands Led to Rubber Gloves," *American Journal of Nursing* 70 (April 1970): 777. Rubber gloves were first used in the surgery of William Stewart Halsted of Johns Hopkins, and he recounted the story himself in "Liature and Suture Material," *Journal of the American Medical Association* 60 (May 13, 1913): 1123.

3. Letter from the archivist at the University of Akron.

4. R. Cautley, G. W. Beebe, and R. L. Dickinson, "Rubber Sheaths as Venereal Disease Prophylactics: The Relation of Quality and Technique to Their Effectiveness," *American Journal of the Medical Sciences* 195 (February, 1938): 155–83.

5. H. E. Butts, "Legal Requirements for Condoms Under the Federal Food, Drug and Cosmetic Act," in M. H. Redford, G. W. Duncan, and D. J. Prager, eds., *The Condom: Increasing Utilization in the United States* (San Francisco: San Francisco Press, 1974).

6. "Condoms of the Wrong Size," in Redford, Duncan, and Praeger, *The Condom*, pp. 289–92.

7. "Update on Condoms—Products, Protection, Promotion," *Population Reports*, Series H, Number 6, (September-October 1982): Volume 10, Number 5.

8. M. Vessy, M. Lawless, and D. Yeates, "Efficacy of Different Contraceptive Methods," *Lancet* 1 (8276) (April 10, 1982): 841–42.

9. W. R. Grady, M. B. Hirsch, N. Keen, and B. Vaughan, *Contraceptive Failure and Continuation among Married Women in the United States, 1970–76.* (Hyattsville, Md.: National Center for Health Statistics, 1981), Working Paper No. 6.

10. *Consumer Reports* 54 (March 1989): 135–42.

9

Sterilization

Voluntary sterilization is the most effective method of contraception known. At the present time, it is also the most widely used method of contraception in the United States. It has become the method of choice for couples who feel they have completed their family and do not want any more children. The major problem with this method is that it is difficult to reverse; those contemplating sterilization should regard it as permanent. One of the choices a couple has is whether the male or the female should be sterilized. There are advantages and disadvantages to either decision.

MALE STERILIZATION

The standard method for sterilizing males is the vasectomy. It is one of the safest, simplest, and most effective methods of contraception available and is widely used in the United States and in Great Britain. It is not so widely used elsewhere although the number of male sterilizations in China and India is very high.

A vasectomy involves cutting into the vas deferens, the excretory duct of the testis, which transports the sperm from each testicle to the prostatic urethra. As indicated in chapter 2, the prostate gland secretes a thin opalescent fluid that carries the sperm manufactured in the testicles. It is the fluid that is visible when ejaculation occurs. The assumption behind the vasectomy is that the passageway of the sperm can be closed by cutting out or blocking a section of the vas deferens.

VASECTOMY

Location of Incision

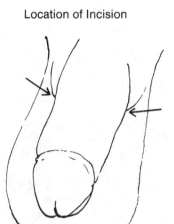

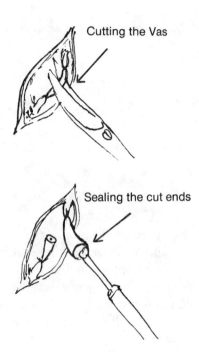

Cutting the Vas

Sealing the cut ends

Illustration by Steven Bullough

It is a comparatively new method of contraception since the importance of the vas deferens was not understood until the nineteenth century. Many of the techniques for performing the operation developed early in the twentieth century when it was used as a method to sterilize patients for eugenic reasons. Criminals, the mentally ill, the retarded, and those with hereditary diseases were often sterilized, many of them involuntarily.[1] In spite of these rather dubious origins of the procedure, it came to be recognized as a legitimate method of voluntary sterilization that was safe, efficient, and relatively inexpensive. It was widely encouraged in India in the 1950s and 1960s where female physicians were scarce and women living in rural areas would not go to a male professional for a pelvic examination, much less sterilization. It was also endorsed and encouraged in the United States by the Association for Voluntary Sterilization.

Vasectomy is a simple, minor surgical procedure, usually performed under local anesthesia, and takes from 10 to 15 minutes to perform. The surgeon makes a small opening in the scrotum, and severs the vas deferens either by tying it, blocking it, or cutting out a small piece. He then repeats the operation on the other side since there are two vasa deferentia, one from each testicle. Some surgeons prefer to make only one incision. Some seal the ends of the vas by ligation (tying it), others by coagulating it with electricity, and still others by using clips.

Regardless of the method, the incision is then closed usually with absorbable sutures such as catgut, although some surgeons make such small incisions that no suturing is required. Postoperative care is relatively simple and involves the patient resting for one or two hours in the clinic and then at home for several more hours. The man should avoid hard work or strenuous exercise for two or three days after surgery and wear a scrotal support for seven or eight days. Sometimes there is mild discomfort, which can be relieved by taking aspirin or other mild painkillers. Usually the incision heals in about a week. Sexual intercourse can be resumed at any time during or after the healing process but contraceptives should continue to be used since infertility is not immediate. In fact, it may take ten weeks or more before the male is infertile. This is because sperm have been stored in the reproductive tract on the urethral side of obstruction and these must be expelled before it is safe to have intercourse without using some other method of contraception. The usual procedure is to have the semen checked for sperm six to eight weeks after the vasectomy; and if they are still present, another check is called for. If sperm continue to be present, after the second check, another surgical procedure might be necessary.

Problems

The major problems with male sterilization seem to be mainly psychological, which is why careful and accurate counseling is essential. A vasectomy is not suitable for men who desire children at a future date because, in most cases, the procedure is not reversible. Those men who equate their masculine image with their ability to impregnate others are not good candidates and should be discouraged from having a vasectomy. In the case of a couple, both partners should agree to the procedure since if one supports the idea while the other still intends to have children, conflict might arise resulting in major marital problems.

There are also some men who, for physical reasons, should not have a vasectomy, at least not right away. The vasectomy should be delayed if there are local skin infections, such as scabies, or genital tract infections that might interfere with the healing of the incision. Physical conditions that might make the operation dangerous or difficult and might count against a vasectomy are varicocele (enlarged veins in the spermatic cord), a large hydrocele (accumulation of fluids in the testes), inguinal hernia (protrusion of the hernial sac containing the intestine through the inguinal opening into the scrotum), filiarsis (a chronic disease caused by the existence of thread worms), and the presence of scar tissue from previous surgery. Some systematic disorders such as diabetes also suggest caution, as does a recent heart attack.

Effectiveness

The failure rate for vasectomy is calculated for every 100 operations, and it is low—about .15 per 100 person-years for those who have an active sex life. This means that there are 15 pregnancies each year for every 10,000 operations. Failures are usually due to four factors:

1. Recanalization of the ends of the vas (the ends grew together naturally) because they were not tied or separated properly. Failure here is due to surgical error.

2. Sexual intercourse took place without contraceptives before the reproductive tract was cleared of sperm.

3. Severing of something else other than the vas. Again, failure is due to surgical error.

4. The rare case where there is more than one vas on one side and the surgeon did not notice this anatomical anomaly. Though this is extremely rare, failure is again due to surgical error.

It is because of the possibility of surgical errors, or engaging in intercourse without a contraceptive before the sperm have disappeared, that sperm testing should be done. In sum, where caution is exercised, both by the physician and the patient, failures should be almost nonexistent.

Before a vasectomy some men worry that their sexual pleasure will be diminished. This is not the case. Ejaculation occurs exactly as it did before the surgery. The only difference is that the fluid contains no sperm.

Possibilities of Reversal

Though our discussion has emphasized that those undergoing vasectomies should regard the procedure as irreversible, this still does not stop some individuals from desiring to reverse the procedure due to unanticipated and unexpected developments, such as remarriage after divorce, the death of one or more children, an improvement in family finances thereby leading to a desire for more children, and the existence of psychological problems associated with vasectomy.

The request rate for reversal of a vasectomy in the United States is low, probably not more than 2 in every 1,000 cases.[2] Still, this adds up to a significant number. Success with the reversal depends both on the condition of the tissue and the skill of the surgeon. The success rate is determined by the ability to impregnate a partner, which at present is about 50 percent. There is, however, a higher rate of success if the ability to ejaculate sperm is the only indicator. Here success has ranged between 80 and 100 percent, and with the development of new techniques it could reach 100 percent. The problem is that vasectomies often lead to decreased sperm counts, which make it less likely that a pregnancy will occur even though a million or even a couple of million sperm are ejaculated. One of the effects of a vasectomy is to encourage the growth of granulomas (benign tumors or growths) in the epididymis (the small oblong body that rests on the posterior part of the testicles), which develop in about 50 percent of vasectomized men. This means that the longer the period between a vasectomy and the attempts at reversal, the smaller the chance of success since the ducts in the epididymis constitute the beginning of the excretory ducts carrying the sperm from the testes. The growth of the granulomas create's obstructions in the ducts making it more difficult for the sperm to pass through. Successful reversals by any measure are nearly 100 percent successful up to two years after the vasectomy, and as high as 91 percent successful for periods of less than ten years, but the dropoff after that is very high.[3]

Other problems also occur, sometimes making restoration difficult. For example, it is possible that the original vasectomy proce-dure damaged nerves in the sheath of the vas that control its rhyth-mic contractions associated with evacuation of the sperm. This would also impede sperm flow. Antibodies to sperm can also be a deterrent to successful reversal. Sperm that are blocked from their normal exit pattern are absorbed by the body and enter the bloodstream where they are interpreted as foreign bodies. Consequently, in some men, antibodies are created to neutralize the sperm. If a reversal is at-tempted, the antibodies move in and neutralize the sperm, reducing fertility. It is for these reasons that reversal is not always successful.

FEMALE STERILIZATION

Methods

Almost all methods of voluntary female sterilization in some way or another block the fallopian tubes that transmit the ova from the

TUBAL LIGATION

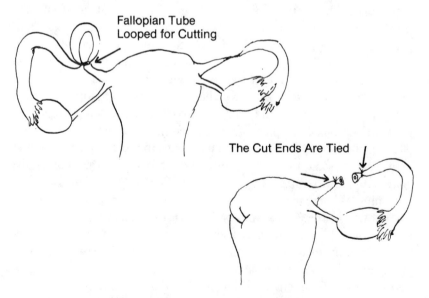

Fallopian Tube
Looped for Cutting

The Cut Ends Are Tied

Illustration by Steven Bullough

ovaries into the uterus. Tying the tubes (tubal ligation) is one of the oldest forms of tubal occlusion. Traditionally it was performed by making a three- to four-inch (10 cm.) incision (a laparotomy) in the abdomen and tying, dividing, resecting, or crushing the tubes, or burying the stumps in the muscular wall of the uterus. Simple ligation (tying off), which dates from 1880, is seldom performed today because of the high failure rate (up to 20 percent), and the most widely used procedures are those involving removal (resection) of a segment of the tube and ligation of the end. There are a number of variations to this method that are of interest to the specialist, but the most widely used technique is the one developed by Ralph Pomeroy who used it early in the twentieth century, although no description of it was published until after his death.[4,5] It is the technique recommended by the International Planned Parenthood Federation Panel of Experts. The procedure involves picking up the tube near the midportion to form a loop, tying (ligating) the base of the loop with an absorbable suture, and cutting off (resecting) the top of the loop. As the suture material is absorbed the ends of the tube pull apart. Failure rate is low (0–0.4 percent), although the rate is higher if the procedure is performed at the time of a Caesarean section, because the tissues are traumatized. The procedure is simple to perform; highly effective; possible in the immediate puerpartum period (the period of 42 days following childbirth); morbidity is low; and, most important for many women, it is potentially reversible.

Since 1960, the procedure has been simplified with the development of the minilaparotomy and laparoscopy. The minilaparotomy, sometimes called the "minilap," can be performed under local anesthesia. A small insertion of about 2.5 cm. (approximately 1 inch) is made. Each fallopian tube is then pulled up into the incision to be cut and tied, blocked with rings or clips, and allowed to slip back into place.

Laparoscopy involves inserting a laparoscope into the abdomen. The incision is smaller than for a minilaparotomy and can be made close to the umbilicus (navel) and thus normally no scar is visible. It is easier, however, to make the incision at a spot somewhat lower in the abdomen since this brings the scope closer to the target organs. The laparoscope is a long tube, somewhat like a telescope, through which the surgeon locates the tubes, severs them, and closes the ends by cautery, clips, or rings.[6]

It is also possible for the surgeon to enter the abdomen through the vagina (a colpotomy), with or without the scope, to carry out the procedures. This approach has been used extensively in India but is less popular in the United States. All of these procedures can be carried out on an outpatient basis under local anesthesia and can be completed in about ten to twenty minutes. If a general anesthetic is used, hospitalization is required and the risk of such surgery is increased substantially because of the inherent risk of such anesthesia.

The Chinese have developed a method of sterilization through chemical occlusion, i.e, by occluding the tubes through chemical burning. This method can be done without surgery and without anesthetic. It involves the insertion of a cannula (a tube) through the cervix and uterus up into the fallopian tubes and the injection of a phenol (carbolic acid) solution. This results in a scarring of the tubes, which ultimately closes the opening. One of the major side effects is mild to moderate pain. Phenol preparations also can cause minor fever, dizziness, nausea, pelvic inflammation, and vaginal discharge. An occasional perforation of the uterus or a peritonitis may occur as well. Chemical occlusion is a very low-cost method of sterilization but it is not reversible.

Experiments are being conducted on two other chemical compounds: quinacrine, a hardening and thickening agent that damages the tissues of the tubal lining, and methyl-cyanoacrylate (MCA), a tissue adhesive that turns from a liquid to a solid when it comes in contact with fluid in the tubes, and thus blocks them.

In order to enhance the possibility of reversal, some surgeons have experimented with various kinds of clips. Failures occasionally occur because of the slippage of the clips, but as new clips have been developed the failure rate has decreased. The so-called spring-loaded clip is the most effective, with a failure rate between 0.2 and 1.5 percent. These can be inserted either through a minilaparotomy or through various vaginal approaches.

The tubal ring is a recent development. It can be installed with a minilaparotomy, a laparoscopy, or through the vagina. A loop of fallopian tube is lifted up and drawn into the cylinder of the applicator, whereupon the ring is slipped onto the base of the loop. The ring then contracts, blocking the tubal opening. Failure rate is as low as 0.3 percent but ranges higher if the ring is inserted immediately following childbirth. Restoring fertility is a high probability when rings have been used.

Problems

One of the dangers of any kind of tubal sterilization is ectopic pregnancy, or the implantation of a fertilized ovum outside the uterine cavity. Though the statistical incidence of this is very low, a substantial percentage of pregnancies in sterilized women are ectopic. Ectopic pregnancies cause severe abdominal pain and require surgical removal.

Women should not undergo sterilization if they have a vaginal or a pelvic infection. But once either of these conditions has cleared up, sterilization may proceed. Women who have had previous pelvic surgery or pelvic infections are likely to have adhesions—scars that cause organs to stick together—that make a minilaparotomy difficult if not impossible and will likely require a regular laparotomy.

Any physical condition that increases the risk of complications during surgery requires special evaluation, and in any case the procedure should only be done in facilities equipped to handle emergencies. Such conditions include heart disease, hypertension or other cardiovascular disease, pelvic masses, uncontrolled diabetes, nutritional deficiences, and umbilical or hiatal hernias.

Although not specifically recommended as a mode of sterilization, any surgical operation that removes essential elements of the reproductive system will result in sterilization. This would include a bilateral oophorectomy (removal of the ovaries), orchiectomy (removal of the testes), or a hysterectomy (removal of the uterus). Ordinarily these operations are carried out because of tumors or other pathology. However, hysterectomies were for a time, and in some cases still are, performed on more women than actually needed them because of some pathology. The fact that these procedures are done less often by the Health Maintenance Organizations (HMOs) than in the fee-for-service sectors continues to document this overutilization. This is because the HMOs bill on a per-head basis, which means they make the greatest profit with fewer procedures while the fee-for-service sector profits from procedures. Hysterectomies are major surgeries, which means the fee to the surgeons is high. Not all unnecessary hysterectomies can be blamed on surgeons, however, since many women may have unconsciously or consciously conspired with the surgeons in this overutilization pattern as a means of being sterilized. One reason for this was that other methods of sterilization were stigmatized and/or not acceptable to religious authorities. The women's movement of the late seventies and eighties helped change the climate of opinion for most Americans, with the possible exception of some devout religious members who regard sterilization as a sin except when a surgeon will connive with a fictitious need to have the uterus removed. Gradually the number of hysterectomies has begun to decline.

Reversibility

Reversal of tubal sterilization is sometimes possible (though a hysterectomy is not). Some surgeons have achieved restorations to the point at which pregnancy rates of 60 percent have been recorded. This number might be somewhat misleading because those surgeons who do not achieve success might not report their results. It is a long, difficult, and costly operation. To reverse the sterilization requires the rejoining of the fallopian tubes in such a way that sperm and ovum can progress in opposite directions through the tubes.

Three factors influence reversibility:

1. the woman's general and reproductive health;

2. the effect of the sterilization procedure on the tubes, including the amount of scarring and the length of the remaining segments; and

3. the technique and skill of the surgeon.

As in the case of men, prognosis becomes poorer the longer the person has been sterilized. Even before deciding to undergo reversal, a basic fertility evaluation test should be done to confirm ovulation. Women over the age of thirty-seven are poor candidates because fertility decreases with age. The fertility of the partner should also be evaluated and entered into the equation.

Reversal is considered major surgery involving microsurgical techniques, and general anesthesia is necessary. This means that the patient should be in good health since major surgery puts a patient at risk. Successful surgery requires that the two segments of the tube must be properly aligned and then sutured (sewn together) without placing stitches through the lumen (or hole). Extreme care also must be taken to prevent adhesions from forming that can kink the tube or impair its mobility.

Though the risk of dying as a result of an operation for sterilization reversal is probably less than 100 per 100,000 women—much less than with many other major surgical procedures—it is much riskier than sterilization itself and far more risky than using temporary contraceptive methods such as oral contraceptives or IUDs. The most serious persistent risk after sterilization reversal is the long-term risk of ectopic pregnancy, which is about ten times more likely in a woman whose tubes have been anastomosized (joined together again) than a woman who had never undergone tubal surgery.

Although some of the current techniques in their experimental stages or in limited use, such as the clamp or the ring, promise greater chance for reattachment than now exists, it is still wise for the person undergoing sterilization to regard it as a permanent condition.

CONCLUSION

Sterilization is emerging as the method of choice for fertility control for those persons who have decided that they have completed their families. In 1987, male sterilization accounted for 13.4 percent of the total contraception in the United States, while female sterilization added another 19.1 percent.[7] When the figures are combined the total is 32.5 percent, which makes sterilization currently the most popular approach to birth control, with oral contraceptives, used by 31.3 percent of the population, the second-ranking approach. The reasons for this trend toward sterilization are many and varied. Sterilization is convenient; sure; and, amortized over time, probably the least expensive method. Many couples worry about conception after the mother is thirty-five or more because of the increased incidence of congenital abnormalities including Down's Syndrome, and yet the average age of menopause is now in the early fifties. This means that the time span of possible fertility is well beyond the optimum years of child bearing. A permanent solution that avoids pregnancy anxiety apparently proves attractive to a large and growing number of people, and probably for this reason the popularity of sterilization can be expected to increase over time among those same segments of the American population.

One of the interesting questions that remains in any discussion of sterilization is why sterilization rates for women remain higher than those for males, especially when sterilization for men is much easier to bring about and less expensive to reverse where reversal is possible. One explanation might well be that women have a greater investment in seeing that they do not become pregnant than men do in seeing that their wives (lovers) do not become pregnant. It might also be that the stigma of being sterilized remains greater for the male than for the female. In any case, like so many other forms of contraception, the answer lies more in the sphere of human psychology than in techniques or in knowledge.

NOTES

1. R. E. Hackett and K. Waterhouse, "Vasectomy Reviewed," *American Journal of Obstetrics and Gynecology* 116 (June 1, 1973): 438–55; A. J. Ochsner, "Surgical Treatment of Habitual Criminals, "*Journal of the American Medical Association* 32 (1899): 867; H. C. Sharp, "Vasectomy as a Means of Preventing Procreation in Defectives," *Journal of the American Medical Association* 53 (1909): 1897–1902.

2. R. D. Amelar and L. Dubin, "Vasectomy Reversal," *Journal of Urology* 121 (May 1979): 547–50.

3. S. J. Silber, "Sperm Granuloma and Reversibility of Vasectomy," *Lancet* 2 (8038) (September 17, 1977): 588–89.

4. E. Bishop and W. F. Nelms, "A Simple Method of Tubal Sterilization," *New York State Journal of Medicine* 39 (1930): 214–16.

5. C. B. Lull, "The Pomeroy Method of Sterilization," *The American Journal of Obstetrics and Gynecology* 59 (1950):1118–23.

6. "Minilaparotomy and Laparoscopy: Safe, Effective, and Widely Used," *Population Reports* Series C, Number 9 (May 1985): Volume 13, p. 125.

7. N. B. Attico, "Contraception Update," *The IHS Primary Care Provider* 14 (July 1989):77–85.

10

Abortion

Abortion is not a form of contraception but it can be construed as a form of birth control, and currently it is probably the most widely used form of birth control in existence. In fact, much of the effort to find more effective forms of contraception has been motivated by a desire to avoid the psychological and physical after-effects of abortion. While legal abortion is one of the safest surgical procedures—with a death rate in the United States of 1.4 per 100,000 procedures, some 11 times safer than a tonsillectomy—illegal abortion kills as many as one woman per 1,000 procedures. This is because complications are greater with illegal abortions.

Some countries, such as Japan and the USSR, tend to rely on abortion instead of contraception as a form of birth control. Legal and inexpensive abortions were adopted by the Japanese in 1948 to combat the overcrowding and poverty following World War II. When contraceptives became more easily available at a later date, Japanese women were reluctant to change their approach. In the Soviet Union, quality contraceptives are still not available and the economic problems are formidable. The abortion ratio in 1988 was 51 percent (the number of abortions compared to the total number of pregnancies times 100).[1] This ratio can be compared with those in countries where contraception is readily available to all segments of the population: e.g., the Netherlands with a rate of 10.7 percent, Great Britain with 16.2 percent, Norway with 17.6 percent, or Sweden with 21.5 percent. The ratio of abortions to pregnancies in the United States is 29.7 percent.[2]

Historically, abortion has been widely used as a method of limiting births, although the methods prescribed were not always effective. For example, a significant portion of the prescriptions in ancient pharmacopeias deal with the concoction of abortifacients, or abortion-causing potions. Methods most often used included drugs, such as ergot, that cause uterine contractions; strong purgatives; douches; and curettage (scraping the uterus with a curette, a spoon-shaped instrument). Various items are also known to have been inserted into the uterus in an attempt to stimulate contractions and cause abortions. In the past, the problem with curettage was the danger of infection and even death; the same problem existed when any object was inserted into the uterus.

Both English common law and Canon (or church) law recognized that inducing abortion before quickening, that is, before the first perceptible movement of the fetus, was not an offense. Abortions in such cases were usually performed by a midwife or a knowledgeable woman, and rarely did men intervene. In the nineteenth century, however, abortion became much more publicized, while scientific research tended to indicate that embryonic development was continuous, with quickening being only one stage. Many Western countries, theoretically in order to protect women from injury, began to enact restrictive abortion legislation. American physicians, in their attempt to gain status over their rivals (such as midwives), also condemned the procedure; their professional societies not only prohibited their members from engaging in abortion, but had such prohibitions enacted into law. All American states, for example, enacted laws prohibiting physicians from performing abortions. The Roman Catholic Church in 1869 eliminated the distinction it traditionally had made between the abortion of a nonanimated and that of an animated fetus (i.e., before and after quickening) and made all abortion murder for the faithful. Western ideas, as they developed in the nineteenth century, also influenced non-Western areas in Africa and Asia; countries in these areas also enacted prohibitions against abortion.

Restrictions and prohibitions, however, did not eliminate the practice. They simply led to the rise of illegal practitioners who operated outside the law. Even when these illegal abortionists were skilled and knowledgeable physicians or midwives (though most were not), they were cut off from hospitals and other facilities that could aid them in the management of emergencies, such as the not infrequent hemorrhaging or infection. In most American states in the twentieth century, the only legal abortions were the so-called therapeutic ones, which were ordinarily allowed only when the pregnancy was diagnosed as dangerous to the mother's life. In the early 1960s there were approximately 8,000 therapeutic abortions a year and an estimated fifty to eighty times as many illegal ones (400,000 to 640,000). This estimate is probably on the low side. A very high maternal mortality rate was associated with these illegal abortions, largely because of bleeding and infection.

As a result, many reformers (especially after the discovery of antibiotics had lessened the dangers of infection) began in the middle of the twentieth century to support the legalization of abortion for the same reason that dedicated reformers had urged that it be made illegal in the nineteenth, namely, to save the lives of pregnant women. The new drive for abortion rights also included the growing recognition of a woman's right to control her own body to the extent that she had a right to decide whether she was going to become or stay pregnant.

Even before the American movement for abortion rights began to grow, other countries had acted. The Soviet Union, for example, had made abortion legal as part of the revolutionary changes introduced in the 1920s. Since abortion in the USSR was used as the major approach to contraception, the numbers escalated rapidly, although the exact figures are not available. In 1936, Stalin, for reasons that are not clear, placed a ban on abortions, which remained in effect until after his death. In 1955, abortions were again permitted. Most of the Soviet bloc countries also legalized abortion in the post–World War II period, as did the Scandinavian countries and Japan.

In America the first real impetus for abortion law reform probably came from the Model Penal Code adopted by the American Law Institute in the 1950s. The proposals were modest, providing for termination of pregnancy when the physical or mental health of the mother was greatly impaired; when the child might be born with a grave physical or mental defect; or when pregnancy resulted from rape, incest, or other felonious intercourse, including illicit intercourse with a girl under the age of sixteen. Gradually, sentiment began to build for changes in the law, and a number of states, including California and Colorado, modified their laws to permit abortion under certain conditions. Similarly, a number of legal cases wound their way through the courts, encouraged by the National Association for the Repeal of Abortion Laws, which was formed in 1969. In 1973, in the case of *Roe* v. *Wade*, the U.S. Supreme Court ruled that abortions were a constitutional right and that laws prohibiting them were null and void, although the rights of states to regulate abortions under certain conditions were recognized. The anonymous Jane Roe, who brought the suit in Texas, was later identified as Norma McCorvey. The decision did not help her since the court procedure took so long that she had already delivered her baby by the time the Supreme Court rendered its decision. In its ruling, the Court held that for the first three months of pregnancy the matter of abortion was to be decided by the woman and her physician. During the next six months the states were permitted to regulate the procedures used in order to assure reasonable standards of care. Only in the last ten weeks, however, could the state ban abortion unless it was necessary to preserve the life of the mother. In spite of various legal challenges that have emphasized the power of the states to regulate abortions, this is essentially the law as this book is being written.

RISKS

When performed by a competent professional under aseptic conditions, abortion is a relatively safe procedure. When performed by inexperienced people or under unhygienic conditions, as so often happens in the case of illegal abortions, it is much more dangerous, not only in terms of maternal deaths, but in terms of long-term complications.

TECHNIQUES

Techniques vary with the stage of fetal development at which an abortion is sought. These can be broken down into early-abortion methods, first-trimester methods, and second-trimester methods.

Early Abortion

Early abortion—sometimes called postcoital contraception, other times menstrual regulation—can be brought about by several methods that rely on hormones or mechanical techniques.

Hormones. Various combinations of the hormones estrogen and progesterone are known to be capable of terminating a pregnancy or bringing about the menses. Though the FDA has not approved any contraceptive for postcoital use, there are effective oral contraceptives for this purpose on the market. The cautious position of the FDA on this matter probably stems more from political considerations than safety concerns. There are many people who consider any contraceptive administered after an unprotected act of intercourse to be an abortifacient.[3] Given this lack of positive approval, there are some clinics, particularly those receiving federal funds, that do not prescribe any postcoital contraception, while other facilities may limit its use to rape victims.

The most commonly used morning-after pill is the oral contraceptive Ovral, which includes 50 micrograms of estrogen and 0.5 milligrams of progestin. A total of four tablets are prescribed in divided doses. The series must start within 72 hours of the incident of unprotected intercourse; preferably, it should start within 24 hours. Although there may be some unpleasant side effects related to this regime—including nausea, vomiting, and breast tenderness—they are much less severe than those experienced with the use of Diethylstilbestrol (DES), the medication of choice in the past for use as a morning-after pill. The effectiveness of the Ovral is, however, comparable.[4]

IUDs. Postcoital insertion of a copper IUD has also proved effective in regulating menses by preventing implantation of the fertilized ovum in the uterus. This method was pioneered by Jack Lippes in the 1970s and involves the insertion of the IUD from one to seven days after the incidence of unprotected intercourse.[5] The use of the IUD has several advantages over DES: since it avoids the side effects, it can be inserted up to seven days after the unprotected intercourse took place, and it affords ongoing protection against further pregnancy if the woman decides to retain the device.

Menstrual Extraction. A third method of bringing about an early abortion is menstrual extraction, which involves the insertion of a *Karman* cannula (tube) into the uterus and the removal of menstrual blood and tissue. A syringe or a suction machine is used to extract the uterine lining. This method, described below, is used for a woman whose period is late; in fact, some women have used it to shorten the length of a menstrual period. No pregnancy test is required but casual use of the technique is *not* recommended since there is a risk of hemorrhage and infection. The method is relatively inexpensive, requires less dilation of the cervix than a suction abortion done at a later point in pregnancy, and, since it is performed without a certain knowledge of pregnancy, it has an advantage for those women who object to the notion of an abortion.

First-Trimester Abortions

Over 90 percent of all abortions take place in the first trimester, after a pregnancy is diagnosed. Two basic techniques are involved: uterine aspiration, sometimes called suction abortion or vacuum aspiration, and dilatation and curettage (D & C).

Uterine Aspiration Technique, or Suction Abortion. This is a comparatively new procedure that originated on a large scale in Asia and came to the West through Soviet and East European sources in the 1960s. It is based, however, on a method pioneered in the nineteenth century by Sir James Young Simpson, who used it to bring on menstruation, hence it is also sometimes called menstrual regulation. Simpson's method was applied to abortions by S. G. Bykov, a Russian, in 1927, and was further perfected in the 1930s by Emil Novak, a Baltimore physician, to bring on menstruation. It was rarely discussed as an abortion technique until 1958, when three Chinese physicians reported on the method in the *Chinese Journal of Obstetrics and Gynecology*.[6] After a urine test to assure that the client is pregnant, blood pressure and pulse are checked, as is blood type. A patient history is also taken emphasizing menstrual, pregnancy, and medical history in order to determine any possible complications that might develop. A pelvic examination is performed to determine the extent of the pregnancy. Then, after emptying her bladder, the patient lies on the table and the medical professional, using a vaginal speculum, exposes the cervix. Both the vagina and cervix are cleaned with an antiseptic solution. The cervix is stabilized by a forcep (or a tenaculum) and dilated. After determining the depth of the uterus, a flexible cannula (tube) with centimeter markings is inserted through the cervix to the full depth of the uterine cavity. Then either a vacuum pump or syringe is used to draw out (aspirate) the inner lining of the uterus, thus bringing out the soft semi-liquid products of conception. The entire aspiration process takes from 45 seconds to 10 minutes depending on the amount that is evacuated (which depends on the length of gestation). Once the process is completed, the cannula is removed and the uterine cavity is further explored with a curette to make sure that it is indeed empty. Patients are then monitored for excessive blood loss, low blood pressure, and pain, and many rest briefly before being discharged. If they are Rh-negative, they are given a *Rhogam* shot to prevent the formation of antibodies. Complications include possible infection or hemorrhage and uterine perforation. Hemorrhage is the most common (in about 1 percent of the cases) but only rarely is the bleeding sufficient to require a transfusion. Uterine perforation is very rare if the operator is experienced, but when it happens it is much more dangerous and often requires surgery. In rare cases a hysterectomy might have to be performed. Abortion-related infection is suspected if fever, abdominal pain, or yellowish vaginal discharge develops within a few days. The infection should be treated with an antibiotic.

Uterine aspiration is the preferred method of first-trimester abortion: since the procedure can be done in a short time, recovery is rapid and complications are few. Uterine aspiration is also relatively inexpensive (under $500) and many health insurance programs cover it.[7]

Dilatation and Curettage. Dilatation and curettage (D & C) is a common gynecological procedure used for taking biopsies to detect malignancies, dealing with prolonged bleeding from the uterus, removing unexpelled placenta after childbirth, making certain that all matter has been expelled after a spontaneous abortion, and inducing abortions. It is an ancient procedure that can be documented from Greek times. The preliminary steps are similar to the aspiration method except that they are usually performed under either a local or general anesthetic. A speculum is inserted into the vagina to expose the cervix, after which the cervix and vagina are cleansed with an antiseptic solution; the cervix is then stabilized and dilated until the opening is large enough to allow the curette to enter and clean out the uterus.

Various techniques can be used to speed up the dilatation process, including the use of laminaria, cervical tampons that swell to three or five times their original diameter when placed in a moist environment. These are usually placed in the cervix at least twelve hours before the curettage takes place. The amount of pain is markedly less than with the metal dilators, and laminaria are particularly helpful in situations where dilatation is difficult, as in the case of the cervix of an immature adolescent or an atrophied cervix. Laminaria are also particularly useful in mid-trimester abortions induced by hypertonic saline or prostaglandins.[8]

Mid-Trimester or Second-Trimester Abortions

Mid-trimester abortions (between the fourth and sixth months) are more difficult. Although both D & C and vacuum aspiration are used early in this three-month period, both become increasingly risky and difficult as pregnancy advances. Clearly the earlier an abortion takes place, the less risk there is to the client, since as the pregnancy progresses there is a higher risk of uterine injury, incomplete abortion, infection, and hemorrhaging. For most second-trimester abortions, a hypertonic saline solution is used.

Hypteronic Saline. This method was first described in 1939 by a Romanian but was not used in the United States or in western Europe until the 1960s. It involves the instillation of hypertonic saline (a 20 percent sodium chloride solution) into the amniotic sac or into the extraovular space (between the amniotic sac and the uterus). The exact mechanism of action is not fully understood but its major effect appears to be an increase in the uterine production and release of prostaglandins, which cause uterine contractions and expulsion of the fetus.[9]

NATURAL PROSTAGLANDINS

Prostaglandins are a group of biologically related fatty acids found in the cardiovascular system, smooth muscles, and other organs. They were discovered half a century ago when a substance was found in human semen that could make smooth muscles, such as those in the uterus, contract or relax. Since it was assumed that the substance was manufactured in the male prostate gland, they were called prostaglandins, although it was later found they were produced in the seminal vesicles as well as other cells. Prostaglandins are effective in inducing abortion at any stage of gestation, and in the form of vaginal suppository have been used within two weeks of a missed period. The most successful use, however, has been in late first-trimester or in second-trimester abortions. Prostaglandins may be administered in a variety of ways including the intra-amniotic and extraovular routes utilized for hypertonic saline. Experimentally, at least, they can also be given intravenously, intramuscularly, intravaginally, orally, or rectally. It is believed that they stimulate cell membrane potentials, create changes in circulatory progesterone levels, and stimulate the myometrium (the muscular wall of the uterus), thus encouraging uterine contractions and expulsion of uterine contents. Aftereffects include nausea, vomiting, and diarrhea.[10]

PROBLEMS AND EFFECTIVENESS

Obviously, abortion is an effective way of planning or spacing births, but it is not a suitable approach for those who have moral objections to the various procedures. Particularly in the case of mid-trimester abortions, there is some risk of death for women with preexisting medical disorders such as sickle cell disease, moderate to severe anemia, cardiac or cardiovascular disorders, and renal disorders, but the risks are not as great for women with those conditions as when they carry a fetus to full term. Abortions performed in the first trimester are much easier and safer than those performed in the second, and are less expensive. Mid-trimester abortions are, however, necessary when there is a late identification of medical disorders that make pregnancy life threatening or when discovery of fetal abnormalities occurs (most often detected by amniocentesis performed after the sixteenth week of gestation). Sometimes ignorance or psychological denial of pregnancy, especially by young women, leads to the putting off of an abortion until the signs and symptoms are obvious. There is also considerable ambivalence about abortion and perhaps even a lack of information on its availability to some people until mid-trimester. Abortions are safest and easiest if they take place in the first trimester.

Effective counseling should be a part of the abortion procedure, particularly for those who face the experience for the first time. Even if they do not subscribe to the teachings of a religion that forbids abortion, many women come to the experience with a great deal of guilt derived from the broader societal norms. Talking about these feelings often helps them to cope. Fear of serious complications or death is also a part of the baggage that most women bring to the abortion experience. Novels and family folklore have traditionally blamed abortions for mysterious deaths and sterility of large numbers of women. Modern movies and soap operas have reinforced this tradition by hinting a fatal abortion to get rid of an unwanted female character. While complications and deaths did occur in significant numbers when the abortionist was an illegal back alley outcast without the support of antibiotics and modern equipment, the death rate was probably never as high as the fictional literature portrayed it. At the present time, an abortion, particularly in the first trimester, is a minor surgical procedure with risks comparable to those of other minor procedures. A realistic appraisal of the actual risk helps put the procedure in perspective.

NOTES

1. "Abortions Outnumber Births in Soviet Union," Reuters quoting the *Moscow News*. *Buffalo News* (November 20, 1989): A-3.

2. E. F. Jones, J. D. Forrest, S. K. Henshaw, J. Silverman, and A. Torres, *Pregnancy, Contraception, and Family Planning Services in Industrialized Countries*. A Study of the Alan Guttmacher Institute (New Haven: Yale University Press, 1989), p. 7.

3. See Lawrence Lader, *Abortion* (Indianapolis, Ind.: Bobbs-Merrill, 1966), and Vern Bullough and Bonnie Bullough, *Sin, Sickness, and Sanity: A History of Sexual Attitudes* (New York: New American Library, 1977), pp. 91-117. R. A. Hatcher, F. Guest, F. Stewart, G. K. Stewart, J. Trus-

sell, S. C. Bowen, and W. Cates. *Contraceptive Technology 1988–1989,* 14th revised edition, (New York: Irvington Publishers, 1988).

4. A. A. Yuzpe. "Postcoital Contraception," *International Journal of Gynaecology Obstetrics* 16 (1979): 497–501. A. A. Yuzpe, R. P. Smith, and A. W. Rademaker, "A Multicenter Clinical Investigation Employing Ethinyl Estradiol Combined with Dl-norgestrel as a Postcoital Contraceptive Agent," *Fertility and Sterility* 37 (1979): 508–13.

5. H. I. Shapiro, *The Birth Control Book* (New York: St. Martin's Press, 1977); H. Lehfeldt, "Choice of Ethinyl Estradiol as a Post-coital Pill," *American Journal of Obstetrics and Gynecology* 116 (1973): 892; A. A. Haspels and R. Andriesse, "The Effect of Large Doses of Estrogen Post Coitum in 2,000 Women," *European Journal of Obstetrical and Gynecological Reproductive Biology* 3 (1973): 113–17.

6. J. Lippes, T. Malik, and H. J. Tatum, "The Post-coital Copper-T," *Advances in Planned Parenthood* 11 (1956): 24–29; J. Lippes, "PID and IUD," paper presented at the World Congress of Gynecology and Obstetrics, Tokyo (October 1979).

7. See, for example, J. Y. Simpson, *Clinical Lectures of the Diseases of Women* (Edinburgh, Scotland: R. Clark, 1872); E. Bykov, "Aspiration of the Gravid Uterus" [in Russian], *Vrachebnoe Delo* 9 (1927): 21; E. Novak, "Suction Curet Apparatus for Endometrial Biopsy," *Journal of the American Medical Association* 104 (1935): 1497; K. T. T'Sai, "Application of Electric Vacuum Suction in Artificial Abortion: 30 Cases" [in Chinese], *Chinese Journal of Obstetrics and Gynecology* 6 (1958): 445; Y. T. Wu and H. C. Wu, "Suction in Artificial Abortion: 300 Cases" [in Chinese], *Chinese Journal of Obstetrics and Gynecology* 6 (1958): 447.

8. "Cervical Dilatation: A Review," *Population Reports*, Series F, Number 6 (September 1977): C. J. Eaton, F. Cohn, and C. C. Bollinger, "Laminaria Tent as a Cervical Dilator Prior to Aspiration-Type Therapeutic Abortion," *Obstetrics and Gynecology* 47 (April 1976): 533–37; Y. Manabe, "Laminaria Tent for Gradual and Safe Cervical Dilatation," *American Journal of Obstetrics and Gynecology* 110 (July 1, 1971): 743–45.

9. T. D. Kerenyi and D. Muzsnai, "Volume and Sodium Concentration Studies in 300 Saline-Induced Abortions," *American Journal of Obstetrics and Gynecology* 121 (March 1, 1975): 590–96.

10. "Pregnancy Termination in Mid-trimester: Review of Major Methods," *Population Reports*, Series F, Number 5 (September 1976).

11

Other Forms of Contraception

This overview of contraceptives aims to be as complete as possible; it is therefore important to mention other contraceptive techniques that do not fall into the generalized categories of the earlier chapters, as well as contraceptives currently under development or soon to be on the market.

SOME TRADITIONAL FORMS

1. Withdrawal or *Coitus Interruptus*

Basically, withdrawal involves the removal of the penis from the vagina prior to ejaculation. The failure rate for this method is high, as much as 23 percent, but this still means that it is better than no protection at all, in which case the pregnancy rate reaches upwards of 90 percent.

One reason for failure is the difference between intentions and actions. Although a couple intends to separate before ejaculation, this goal is not always achieved for a variety of physiological and psychological reasons.

A second reason has to do with a basic aspect of physiology, namely, the existence of Cowper's glands. These are located just below the seminal vesicles; when a male becomes aroused these glands secrete a fluid that appears as clear, slippery droplets at the opening of the penis. Sometimes the fluid contains sperm, which means that even before ejaculation, sperm can dribble from the penis.

2. *Coitus Reservatus*

This is a method often associated with secret rituals and rites of ancient China and India. In these ancient societies there was a belief that too great a loss of *yang,* the male's seminal essence excreted at ejaculation, would lessen a man's vigor and make him less able to have male descendants. The way to avoid this was to have intercourse until the women had her orgasm, and thus gain some of her *yin* essence, but then not ejaculate. The male was to keep his penis in the vagina but not ejaculate, leaving it there until the erection had passed. For those unable to train themselves mentally to control their ejaculation, the Taoist teachers (Tao is an ancient Chinese religion) taught the male to exert pressure with his finger on the urethra between the scrotum and the anus. This would prevent the ejaculation of semen, diverting it into the bladder where it would be excreted with the urine. The Taoists, lacking an understanding of modern physiology, held that the semen ascended upward to the brain where it served as a rejuvenating force for the body. Similar ideas appear in Indian tantrism.[1] This method of contraception was also used among the Oneida community established by John Humphrey Noyes in upstate New York in the middle of the nineteenth century. Noyes called it "male continence," which he explained as the art of prolonging the act of intercourse without ejaculation.

Though both more physiologically and psychologically difficult to practice than withdrawal, the results of *coitus reservatus* would probably be the same, although the prolonged intercourse with *coitus reservatus* allows slightly more seepage of semen.

3. Postcoital Douching

There is a widespread belief that douching with an acidic solution of vinegar and water or citric acid (lemon juice) and water will have a contraceptive effect. Though it is true that acidic solutions do in fact kill sperm, the problem is to make certain that the solution comes in contact with the sperm, and this is difficult to do with douching. Sperm start swimming through the cervix and into the uterus in a matter of seconds after ejaculation; even if a woman has an acidic douche ready to insert into her vagina immediately after the male withdraws, many sperm may have escaped to the safety of the uterus.

Though failure rate with acidic douches is high (40 per 100 woman-years), they are certainly better than nothing.[2] Less effective are douches popular with some teenagers, such as cola and similar beverages (shaking the bottle propels the fluid into the vagina). Unfortunately, cola has no spermicidal properties and the sugar content can trigger the development of a yeast infection.

4. Plastic Wrap and Similar Barriers

Since some adolescents know about the importance of erecting a barrier between the cervix and the entrance of the sperm, various devices have been tried other than the standard barriers of diaphragm, cap, or condom. One frequently reported to clinics is plastic wrap. Sad to report, this clingy material is not effective since it does not stay in place effectively and does not fit tight enough to prevent the entrance of sperm.

5. Breast-Feeding

Because breast-feeding delays the onset of menstruation, it has often been regarded as a short-term form of contraceptive. Studies in developing countries show that mothers who breast-feed for an extended period do not begin menstruating until an average of ten months after delivery as compared with three months for mothers who do not breast-feed for a long period. It also takes them longer to conceive a child after their most recent birth.[3] Though the correlation with breast-feeding and delay in conception is well documented, it is not always clear how much of this delay is due to the physiological effects of breast-feeding, because in some cultures intercourse with nursing mothers is frowned upon. This in itself would have considerable contraceptive effect. The onset of menstruation even with lactating women is also closely associated with levels of nutrition and physical well-being. For example, a study of Bostonian and Taiwanese women who breast-fed for one to six months, indicated that a higher proportion of the Boston women had begun to menstruate within six months than the women from Taiwan.[4] It is also important to note that ovulation begins before menstruation, although in many women the first cycle is anovulatory (not fertile). In sum, the best advice for women who are breast-feeding and who are also engaging in sexual intercourse is to use one of the contraceptive methods discussed earlier. If a diaphragm or cap is being used, these devices should be refitted after the birth of the baby.

THE CONTRACEPTIVE VALUE OF OTHER FORMS OF SEXUAL INTERCOURSE

Obviously, to become pregnant it is necessary to bring the sperm into contact with the egg and this cannot be done if sexual intercourse involves other orifices than the vagina.

1. Anal Intercourse

Historically, one of the ways in which individuals have avoided becoming pregnant is through anal intercourse, the pentration of the anus by the penis. Since the anus is rich in nerve endings and is involved in the sexual response whether or not it is directly stimulated, some people enjoy this form of intercourse. The anus does not lubricate very well and some form of lubrication has to be provided such as K-Y jelly or other forms of sterile, water soluble solutions. Petroleum-based lubricants should not be used in the rectum, or for that matter in the vagina, because they tend to accumulate and are not as easily discharged as those that are water soluble. Oil-based lubricants also weaken barrier contraceptive devices, including the condom.

The anal sphincter responds to penetration with an initial contraction that may be uncomfortable. In a tense, inexperienced person, the contraction may last for a minute or longer while those experienced in this form of intercourse appear to relax much more quickly and the spasm lasts less than thirty seconds. Usually when the spasm has run its course, the discomfort disappears. Masters and Johnson, in their studies of the sexual response, found that in 11 of 14 episodes involving penetration of a female by a male, the female had an orgasm.[5] Heterosexual couples who engage in anal intercourse should be cautioned, however, that vaginal intercourse ought not to be started immediately after anal sex. The penis should be thoroughly washed first. The anus contains bacteria that can cause infection if introduced into the vagina.

2. Oral-Genital Sex

Oral-genital sex is fairly common in erotic foreplay but some couples also use it to reach orgasm. Technically, *cunnilingus* (oral stimulation of the female genitals) and *fellatio* (oral stimulation of the male genitals) can be performed in a variety of ways and in various positions. Often the couple takes turns stimulating one another; other couples prefer simultaneous oral stimulation. The latter procedure is popularly known as the *soixante-neuf* or "69." Many couples enjoy having various parts of their body massaged, kissed, licked, sucked, or gently nibbled. Couples have to learn what techniques are erotically arousing. A word of caution, however, is necessary when engaging in cunnilingus. Air should not be blown into the vagina; it can enter the abdominal cavity through the fallopian tubes and cause infection.

Obviously, if erotic stimulation can suffice without penile-vaginal contact, pregnancy will not occur.

3. Mutual Masturbation

Masturbation is the most common form of sexual outlet for many Americans. Usually it is done alone and for this reason is sometimes called autoeroticism, the seeking of pleasure with oneself. Mutual masturbation involves a couple together: in general, this involves the partners focusing on each other's genitals. The most sensitive areas of the penis are the glans or tip, the frenulum on the underside of the glans, the shaft, and the scrotum. The female is more complicated. Masters and Johnson, for example, found that none of their female research volunteers masturbated in quite the same way.[6] Other researchers have supported this finding. Most women preferred to stimulate the entire genital area, including the inner lips of the vagina and the clitoris. The clitoral gland is very sensitive and direct stimulation for an extended period of time can be very irritating. Mutual masturbation involves effective communication between partners as to what they most enjoy. Oral-genital stimulation is often involved in mutual masturbation as is a great deal of touching and feeling elsewhere on the body. Ordinarily, mutual masturbation does not result in pregnancy. The reason the word "ordinarily" is used here is because strange events have been reported, including the tale of a woman who claimed that her pregnancy followed a bath in a tub used by her masturbating husband. Most such events can be discounted, but if ejaculation does take place, care should be taken that no portion of the semen is transmitted to the vagina by the hands of the partner or by other means.

WHAT DOES THE FUTURE HOLD?

Several contraceptive methods or improvements on old ones are being readied for the market.

1. RU 486

The antiprogestin mifepristone (RU 486) was developed by the French pharmaceutical firm Roussel-Uclaf with an academic team under the direction of Étienne-Émile Baulieu. Though anti-abortionists in the United States labeled RU 486 the "French death pill" and in 1988 threatened boycotts that temporarily forced Roussel-Uclaf to stop research,[7] French government pressure encouraged the firm to continue. RU 486 works by blocking the normal action of the hormone progesterone during pregnancy, thus preventing the endometrium from accepting or keeping the implantation of the embryo. It can be used to induce early nonsurgical abortions or it can be administered routinely each month just before menstruation is due. The dose is not yet firmly established but it usually involves taking a pill for four days just before the onset of the menses. Used in this way it might be termed a menstrual regulator since the woman would not know whether or not she was pregnant. Dizziness, severe cramps, and heavy bleeding have been reported, typical of a spontaneous abortion. This particular pill is also not yet 100 percent effective, and in perhaps as many as 20 percent of the cases where pregnancy has taken place curettage is necessary to complete the termination. The effects of the pill on an exposed fetus of a woman who did not know she was pregnant are unknown. Chemical abortifacients such as RU 486 also carry the danger that an ectopic pregnancy may be overlooked. At present the drug is also expensive.

Though some have talked of preventing it from ever being available in the United States, this seems unlikely since RU 486 has many more uses than menstrual regulation. At present it is believed that

RU 486 is effective against Cushing's syndrome, a condition resulting from an excess production of cortisone. It apparently will also help in the treatment of burns and abrasions, and against the spread of breast cancer. RU 486 also has potential for being used as a conventional contraceptive since it may prevent ovulation.[8]

The demonstrations against the morality of using RU 486 probably attest more to the growth in the anti-choice movement than to the immorality of employing the compound. Its primary action, when taken before the menses, is to dislodge (or prevent the implantation of) the blastocyte (the cell mass that develops a few days after fertilization) from the uterus. RU 486 would, however, make the termination of an early pregnancy a more private matter because the pill could be taken at home and this would serve as a deterrent to effective demonstrations and political action against women who chose to abort. Moreover, the public outcry by the anti-choice forces has been effective because, as of this writing, neither the French company, Roussel-Uclaf, nor any American pharmaceutical company has applied to the Food and Drug Administration for permission to market the product in United States.

2. Depo-Provera

Depo-Provera is an injectable progestin compound widely used outside of the United States. The World Health Organization (WHO) and seventy foreign governments have decided that this contraceptive is safe enough for broad use. A single injection can stop ovulation for three months and the short-term side effects are regarded as minor. It is manufactured by the Upjohn Company, which requested FDA approval though it has thus far been rejected. The FDA panel concluded that the contraceptive is neither safe nor unsafe. One of the points of controversy was that Depo-Provera caused high incidence of breast cancer in both dogs and monkeys. Upjohn argued that women respond differently than dogs or monkeys to the progestin in Depo-Provera and that the doses in animals were far higher than those given to humans, sometimes as much as 50 percent higher. The panel did not accept this argument, although, interestingly, the drug is currently approved in the United States for the treatment of endometrial cancer.[9] Upjohn has presently withdrawn its application for FDA approval, but if it continues to be effective throughout the world, Depo-Provera will ultimately enter the U.S. market.

Some of the hesitation on the part of the FDA may also be related to the history of progestins. In years past they were used during pregnancy to prevent spontaneous abortions. However, their use caused a high incidence of birth defects, which might not have been caused by progestins so much but may well have been the result of the drug's ability to prevent the loss of a fetus that was already abnormal. Current research is not clear on this point.[10]

3. Male Contraceptives

Researchers in the United States and elsewhere have long been seeking an effective, easy to use, coitally independent, reversible contraceptive for men. Research is concentrated on either hormonal suppression of sperm production or chemical interference at the sites of sperm production.

Hormonal Suppression of Sperm Production. One such product is based upon an analogue of luteinizing-hormone releasing hormone (LHRH), produced in the hypothalamus, one of the control substances that signals the pituitary gland to stimulate the testes to release testosterone and other steroid hormones necessary for sperm production. Thus far, a major difficulty with the drugs that act like LHRH is that by suppressing testosterone production, they also suppress the male libido and potency as well as affecting secondary sex characteristics (such as beard and breasts). To counteract this, another hormone, usually a testosterone-based one, must be taken.[11]

Steroid Hormones. Androgens (male sex hormones), and two types of female sex hormones, progestins and estrogens, inhibit production in men of the pituitary hormones that control sperm production. Most promising are androgens given alone or combined with progestin. Two major problems remain: (1) complete sperm suppression cannot be achieved in all men, and (2) the testosterone compounds tested so far must be given as weekly injections. Animal studies are continuing. One compound, testosterone enanthate (TE), is being tested at the University of Washington where injections reduce sperm production to zero while the male is receiving injections and return to normal when injections are stopped.[12] It is now in the process of being tested on a larger scale.

Inhibin. Inhibin is a peptide (an amino acid-protein compound), produced in the testes, that inhibits release of follicle stimulating hormone (FSH), the pituitary hormone. Though theoretically it should suppress sperm production without affecting testosterone secretion, thus maintaining libido and potency, Inhibin was only isolated and its basic structure identified in 1985. Work is now underway, using recombinant DNA technology, to produce large enough quantities to test it in animals.[13]

Chemical Interference with Sperm Production. The major breakthrough in this area is Gossypol, which works by inhibiting an enzyme that has a crucial role in the metabolism of sperm and the cells that make sperm. It was first identified as an antifertility agent as a result of some studies in China in the 1950s growing out of an effort to explain extremely low birth-rates in a particular geographic area. The phenomenon of low birth-rate was eventually related to the residents' exclusive use of crude cottonseed oil for cooking. Further investigation revealed that the active substance was Gossypol, a phenol compound found in the seed, stem, and roots of the cotton plant. Clinical trials of Gossypol began in 1972 in China but two problems emerged in the long-term studies. (1) Some men developed hypokalemia (low potassium concentration in the blood), which might be remedied by administration of potassium. (2) More importantly, sperm production in some men did not resume when they stopped taking Gossypol. Present research is focused on finding a nontoxic component of Gossypol, or a drug similar to it, that would be effective and reversible.[14]

Temporary Vasectomy. A nonchemical intraluminal device that creates a "temporary vasectomy" is being explored. The device can be removed readily when fertility is desired. Clinical trials in the United States have not yet begun.[15]

4. Vaginal Rings

Levonorgestrel Rings. The World Health Organization and the Population Council continue to study the silastic vaginal ring and predict worldwide availability in the mid-1990s. Worn around the cervix, the ring releases levonorgestral, a synthetic hormone of the progestin family, which makes the cervical mucus virtually impregnable to sperm. The ring is designed to stay in place for three weeks whereupon the woman removes it for a week during menses and then reinserts it. The same ring can be used for three months. Present studies indicate a pregnancy rate of 3.5 per 100 woman-years. The ring has caused irregular bleeding, which accounts for the number of women who discontinued its use. The ring also resulted in some irritation and infection and it can be accidentally expelled, particularly when women squat to defecate, as they often do in many Third World countries.

Progesterone Ring. This is a similar ring containing the natural hormone progesterone. It is designed especially for breast-feeding women so they will not be exposed to synthetic hormones that might affect the composition or quantity of their breast milk. It can remain in the vagina for three months. The ring has the same side effects as levonorgestrel in that bleeding or spotting often occurs, as does irritation and infection.

Combination Rings. These include a mixture of hormones such as levonorgestrel and an estrogen compound, which virtually eliminates ovulation, though the same problems exist.[16]

5. Progestin Implants

Currently available in Scandinavian countries, Indonesia, and South America are silastic polymer-based rods or capsules (Norplant), which when inserted under the skin, slowly release a form of progestin that acts on the hypothalamus and pituitary to suppress the luteinizing-hormone (LH) surge causing ovulation. Implants provide long-term contraceptive protection. Norplant comes in one of two forms: either with six hollow silastic (silicone rubber) capsules or two solid silastic rods. The first is effective for five years, the second for three. The

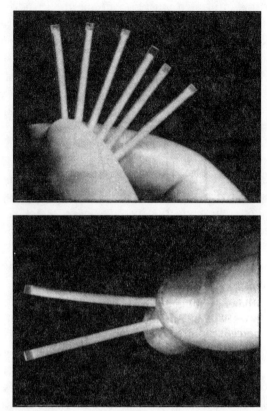

Norplant implants release the progestin levonorgestrel. They are inserted just under the skin in the arm. The 6-capsule system (top) provides almost complete protection from pregnancy for five years. Norplant-2 (bottom), using two rods, is effective for at least three years.

Photograph courtesy of Population Reports.

capsules and rods were developed in the United States but are currently manufactured in Finland. Wyeth Laboratories has requested permission to introduce it into the United States. The six capsules or two rods are implanted just under the skin along the inside of the upper or lower arm. The best time to insert them is when a woman is menstruating but certainly not later than five to seven days after the menses have begun. This ensures that the woman is not pregnant. The skin is infiltrated with a local anesthetic (lidocaine) where the implant is to take place and then a small incision about an inch long is made and the capsules are implanted in an operation that lasts about ten minutes. The incision is then covered with a dressing for three to five days. Insertion is not particularly painful for most women, although the area may be bruised and sore for several days. For some women the implant may be visible. Removal of the implant is more difficult than insertion; the same procedure is used but it takes a little longer to locate and extract the implants. If there is not much swelling or trauma, the new capsule or rod can be inserted to replace the old one. The implants release levonorgestrel (the progestin in several popular brands of oral contraceptives).

The implants eliminate the inconvenience of taking pills, positioning devices, or inserting spermicides. They are also less expensive than oral contraceptives and release hormones at a regular, even interval. Since they contain no estrogen, implants do not have any cardiovascular side effects. Infertility is reversed by removing the implants; in fact, all study patients ovulated within seven weeks after the implants were removed. No effect on breast-fed infants' hormone levels was found.

Effectiveness. Norplant provides almost complete protection against pregnancy. Its failure rate is less than one per 100 woman-years, which makes Norplant as effective as oral contraceptives and intrauterine devices. Effectiveness decreases slightly after five years, and replacement at that time is recommended. Norplant two, or the rod system, is not quite as effective or as long-lasting, and it is recommended that these be replaced every three years.

Side Effects. There are few side effects apart from menstrual changes. Many women report excessive, prolonged, or irregular vaginal bleeding when the implants are first inserted but the bleeding diminishes after a time. There has been a study in which Norplant users reported more headaches than normal. Later, if the woman does decide to become pregnant, she has to have the implant surgically removed. Norplant implants should enter the American market in the 1990s.

Biodegradable Implants. Biodegradable implants, which deliver progestins from a capsule or pellet that gradually dissolves in body tissues, are currently undergoing experimental trials. Two types of these implants are being tested: (1) a polymer capsule filled with a progestin and (2) pellets consisting of the progestin norethindrone and small amounts of cholesterol. The first, called Carpornor, was developed by the Research Triangle Institute in North Carolina. Inserted under the skin of the arm or the hip, it is effective for 18 to 24 months, after which it begins to biodegrade. It releases hormone much faster than the silastic capsule and thus requires a higher storage dose. Few side effects have been reported in preliminary trials, although the average length of the menstrual cycle was about four days shorter than before the device was inserted.

The progestin and cholesterol pellets were developed by Gopi Gupta while working at the Population Council. A four-pellet regime seems to work for as long as a year, during which ovulation ceases. Of the women who used the pellets more than half experienced irregular menstrual patterns accompanied by bleeding or spotting between periods. Amenorrhea (abnormal absence of menstrual flow) occurred in 14 percent of the women within six months. The pellets relieved moderate and even severe menstrual pain in most women who had previously experienced it. Trials are still being carried out.[17]

6. Injectables

At present over eighty countries use various injectables, including Depo-Provera, but none have been approved for contraceptive use in the United States. In addition to Depo-Provera, made by Upjohn, injectables would also include Noristerat, a progestin injection made by Schering, and progestin/estrogen combinations that are currently under study. These long-acting injectables are highly effective for the three-month period for which they are designed. Both the Upjohn and the Schering products are widely used outside of the United States.

In addition to these there are injectable microspheres and microcapsules that consist of a biodegradable shell and one or more hormones, which are released in a manner similar to that of implants. Depending on the formulation, a single injection can provide contraception for one, three, or six months. Once administered they cannot be removed, although they ultimately disintegrate in the body. These microspheres and microcapsules contain a progestin. They have some of the same side effects as the implants and are about as effective. Microspheres seem to lessen the large initial burst of hormone that occurs with the microcapsule. They seem to be very effective, and in China, where monthly injections of microcapsules have been tested, the pregnancy rate was about 1.1 per 100 woman-years. Considerable testing still needs to be done and the research is not as far along as for the implants.[18]

7. Antipregnancy Vaccine

Here research is in an early phase. Thus far such vaccines have been tested mainly on baboons and chimpanzees. Current results indicate that the vaccines stimulate production of antibodies against the chorionic gonadotropin (GT) hormone that supports the implantation of a fertilized egg. If the GT hormone is blocked, pregnancy cannot occur.[19]

8. Electric Contraceptives

Patented in 1986 was a cyclindrical device three-quarters of an inch long and a quarter of an inch in diameter which, when placed inside the cervical canal, creates a weak electrical field (about .5 milliamperes) in the cervical mucus. The charge is imperceptible to the wearer of the device but it immobilizes sperm at the entrance to the canal. The device was invented by Steven Kaali, a gynecologist and obstetrician in Dobbs Ferry, New York, but it is not clear how the mechanism works. As of this writing it is still being tested.[20]

NOTES

1. Vern L. Bullough, *Sexual Variance in Society and History* (Chicago: University of Chicago Press, 1976), pp. 245–316.

2. Leonide Martin, *Health Care of Women* (Philadelphia: J. B. Lippincott, 1978), p. 60.

3. J. Knodel and H. Kitchner, "The Impact of Breast Feeding on the Biometric Analysis of Infant Mortality," *Demography* 14 (1977): 391–409.

4. G. S. Masnick, "The Demographic Impact of Breast Feeding: A Critical Review," *Human Biology* 51 (1979): 109–25.

5. W. H. Masters and V. E. Johnson, *Homosexuality in Perspective* (Boston: Little Brown and Company, 1979).

6. W. H. Masters and V. E. Johnson, *Human Sexual Response* (Boston: Little Brown and Company, 1966).

7. G. Kolata, "Boycott Threat Blocking Sale of Abortion-Inducing Drug," *New York Times* (February 22, 1988): p. 1.

8. Joseph Palca, "The Pill of Choice," *Science* 245 (September 22, 1989): 1319–23, and Jeremy Cherfas, "Étienne-Émile Baulieu: In the Eye of the Storm," *Science* 245 (September 22, 1989): 1323–24.

9. Marjorie Sun, "Panel Says Depo-Provera Not Proved Safe," *Science* 226 (November 22, 1984): 950–51.

10. *Physician's Desk Reference,* 39th ed. (Mahopac, N.Y.: Edward R. Barnhart, 1985), pp. 2109–10.

11. S. Bhasin, T. J. Fielder, and R. S. Swerdloff, "Dissociating Anti-fertility Effects of a GnRH Antagonist from Its Adverse Effects on Mating Behavior: The Critical Importance of Testosterone Dose," in G. I. Zatuchni, A. Goldsmith, I. M. Spieler, and J. J. Sciarra, eds., *Male Contraception: Advances and Future Prospects* (Philadelphia: Harper & Row, 1986), pp. 329–35.

12. D. H. Lewis, T. R. Tice, and L. R. Beck, "Overview of Controlled Release Systems for Male Contraception," in Zatuchni, Goldsmith, Spieler, and Sciarra, *Male Contraception,* pp. 336–46. See also L. G. Blanchard, "Birth Control Breakthrough?" *The Washington Alumnus* (Autumn 1989): 14–16.

13. "Research on New Male Contraceptive Methods, "*Population Reports,* Series 1, Number 33 (November-December 1986): Volume 14, Number 5, J–902.

14. Thomas H. Maugh II, "Male 'Pill' Blocks Sperm Enzyme," *Science* 212 (April 17, 1981): 314; B. H. Vickery, M. B. Griff, J. C. Goodpasture, K. K. Bergström, and K. A. M. Walker, "Toward a Same-Day Orally Administered Male Contraceptive," in Zatuchni, Goldsmith, Spieler, and Sciarra, *Male Contraception,* pp. 271–97.

15. Ibid., pp. 183-207, 227-50.

16. "Hormonal Contraception: New Long-Acting Methods," *Population Reports,* Series K, Number 3 (March–April 1987): Volume 16, Number 1, K68–69.

17. Ibid.

18. Ibid., K66–68.

19. "Contraceptives: On Hold," *Newsweek* (May 5, 1986):68.

20. Tom Dworetzky, "Here's a Shocker: A Contraceptive wth Electric Potential," *Discover* (January 1987):16.

12

Contraception:
Recommendations and Conclusions

The choice of a method of birth control involves four major considerations: (1) the effectiveness of the method, (2) its side effects, (3) personal preference, and (4) the method's potential for disease prevention.

EFFECTIVENESS

Throughout this book the effectiveness of each method has been discussed in terms of the Pearl index (failures per 100 woman-years of exposure). The data used to calculate this index are assumed to include studies of both long-term and short-term users. Another way of determining the effectiveness of a given method is to examine the rate of failures over the first year of use. This comparison could be the most useful approach for those readers who are just beginning to use contraception. Table 1 utilizes this approach for the more common contraceptives. Two different failure rates are shown: the rate that would be expected if the users followed directions carefully, were well instructed in the method, and were carefully supervised; and the failure rate that is seen when ordinary people use the method without such care, planning, and supervision.

Notice the wide differences with some methods between the failures experienced by those in the first group and the more ordinary user

TABLE 1
FIRST YEAR FAILURE RATES OF
COMMON BIRTH CONTROL METHODS[1]

Method	Expected Failure Rate (%)	Typical Failure Rate (%)
Sterilization		
tubal ligation	0.4	0.4
vasectomy	0.15	0.15
Injectable Progestin	0.3	0.3
Oral Contraceptives		
combined	0.1	2.0
multiphasic	0.5	3.0
IUD (nonmedicated)	1.0	2.0
Condom	2.0	12.0
Diaphragm & spermicide	3.0	18.0
Cervical cap & spermicide	5.0	18.0
Sponge (nulliparous women)	14.0	18.0
Spermicides	5.0	21.0
Natural family planning	8.0	20.0
Early withdrawal	7.0	18.0
Douche	20.0	40.0
Chance	90.0	90.0

in the second group. The methods with the greater differences tend to be the ones in which there is heavy participation by the user, including the barrier methods, natural family planning, and withdrawal. However, even the pill shows a difference since the expected failure rate is close to zero and pill users who forget an occasional pill bring the number to two or three per 100 woman-years.

SIDE EFFECTS

The side effects of most of the current popular methods have been reduced by research. The oral contraceptives, which once had significant side effects, have been greatly improved so that now the only persons with any significant risk for heart and blood vessel problems are older women who smoke. In certain women IUDs can increase the possibility of infection or cause heavy menstrual bleeding. Women who have frequent bladder infections may irritate their bladders if they use a diaphragm. However, to put these side effects in perspective, it is important to remember that none of the methods of birth control, including a first-trimester abortion, is as dangerous as a full-term pregnancy.[2]

PERSONAL PREFERENCE

Personal preference and a careful self-assessment of the strengths and weaknesses of the user can be important in the selection of a birth control method. People who forget to take pills or cannot remember to put in a diaphragm before having sex may be better off with one of the more permanent methods such as an IUD or injectable progestin when it becomes available in the United States. Women who have good memories, and do not want to be bothered with a barrier method, often choose oral contraceptives; and they can continue using them well into their thirties if they do not smoke. For people who are finished having a family, sterilization of one of the partners is emerging as the most popular approach. Natural family planning methods are complex, but dedicated, conscientious users are achieving significant control over fertility. Each individual will want to think through the options that best fit his or her personality, belief system, and preference.

DISEASE PREVENTION

Because of the current increase in the danger of sexually transmitted diseases, particularly AIDS, the potential for preventing the spread of disease is becoming an important variable in contraceptive choice. The condom, which was a favored contraceptive in an earlier era, has again become very popular. In an article published in the *Journal of Sex Research,* Ira Reiss and Robert Leik discussed the two major strategies that have been proposed to stem the tide of the AIDS epidemic. They review a brochure from the Surgeon General, which was sent to every U.S. household in 1988, advising people to limit sexual contacts to "one mutually faithful, uninfected partner."[3] Reiss and Leik suggest that this is a futile approach because the average partner has already had more than one sexual mate, and early infection with the Human Immunodeficiency Virus (HIV) produces no symptoms. It is virtually impossible for an ordinary observer to identify the AIDS carrier. They argue that everyone should use condoms with a spermicide for *every* sexual encounter, and that this is the only way to stop the AIDS epidemic that is now raging. Their point of view is supported by impressive mathematical calculations.[4] The reader is urged to consider it seriously and at the very least use a barrier contraceptive for any casual sexual encounter.

THE RESEARCH FRONTIER

In 1970, Carl Djerassi, who developed the synthetic estrogen used in the modern contraceptive pill, wrote an article on what would happen in the field of contraception in 1984.[5] He predicted that birth control in the 1980s would not differ much from that in 1970 since the lead time for development was so great. His prediction was accurate. What he said about the eighties is also true of the nineties. Probably all the contraceptives mentioned in this book will still be on the market by the end of the century, though they might appear under different trade names.

Djerassi, who once again surveyed the contraceptive field in 1989, was much more pessimistic than he had been earlier, particularly because he felt that the United States was falling behind in contraceptive research. He argued that this was due to three major factors: (1) the stringent animal toxicology tests demanded by the FDA after 1969 in response to concern over long-term effects of contraceptives; (2) the impact of congressional hearings, particularly those held by Senator Gaylord Nelson early in 1970, and the subsequent disaster of the Dalkon Shield IUD; and (3) the litigious character of American society during the past two decades, especially where drugs and medical practice are concerned.[6]

Though there is considerable truth in what Djerassi said, it could also be argued that Americans traditionally have been ambivalent about contraceptives and that there have been cycles of greater and lesser research on the technology of contraception. One of the basic deterrents to the development of better birth control methods in America is the fact that during the past three decades fertility research has been dominated by the pharmaceutical industry. This is true even in America's universities where industry grants are vigorously sought. As one would expect, drug companies spend their developmental money to increase profits, not to seek basic scientific knowledge or to solve societal problems, although if this also happens so much the better. There are some tried and true oral contraceptives on the market that bring in a good return each year so new research is not a high priority, although reformulation and repackaging of existing products certainly is. New types of male contraceptives are not the highest priority, because women are the people who become pregnant and who are most motivated to buy contraceptive material. The recent improvement in the quality control of condoms is related to the AIDS epidemic and not to the need for better contraception.

Both the federal Food and Drug Administration's demand for more effective testing and the congressional response to the Dalkon Shield incident came about because of the failure of the pharmaceutical industry to police itself. Before malpractice litigation became so popular in the United States, some drug companies were much more willing to market products after only minimal testing and, in the case of the Dalkon Shield, allegedly to even use fraudulent data.

Though there was some discussion of the Dalkon Shield in the chapter on IUDs, the case is such a pivotal one in the marketing and sale of contraceptives that it deserves to be restated as an illustration of the difficulties that can occur when the greed for profits sweeps away the need for effective research. The initial problem started with the actions of Hugh J. Davis, then a faculty member at the School of Hygiene and Public Health at Johns Hopkins University. According to Morton Mintz, a reporter for the *Washington Post*, who covered federal regulatory agencies, Davis allegedly invented the shield, produced false and misleading test results, and earned royalties on every shield sold, all while passing himself off in medical journals, books, and congressional testimony as an impartial expert. A second villain, according to Mintz, was Ellen Preston, a pediatrician, and A. H. Robins's liaison with physicians, who was allegedly totally unconcerned about the mounting toll of injuries and deaths reported to her by other physicians. Still another villain, according to Mintz,

was the management of the A. H. Robins Company who, throughout
the controversy, showed far more interest in profit than in preventing
further deaths and injuries. Company officials allegedly destroyed
documents and made a policy of misleading both physicians and the
federal government when responding to questions about the shield.
When one employee, upon discovering that the shield's design encouraged the growth of bacteria along the tail of the device and
facilitated their entry into the uterus, recommended a simple solution,
he was not only ignored but reprimanded and forced out of his job.
The net result was that as claims mounted, the company, after more
than 4.5 million shields were sold at considerable profit, finally suspended marketing in the United States. Ultimately, $395 million in
legal judgments and settlements were awarded against A. H. Robins,
forcing it to declare bankruptcy in 1985.[7] Unfortunately, the pharmaceutical company of G. D. Searle, fearing a similar fate, began taking
its widely used copper-7 IUD off the market at the beginning of
1986; this withdrawal left millions of American women with a narrow
range of alternatives, since for a time no IUD was available. The
famous Lippes Loop had been taken off the market, due to declining
sales and profits in the United States, though it remained in use
throughout much of the rest of the world.

Though the temporary loss of the IUD in America's arsenal of
contraceptive techniques is to be deeply regretted, it is hard to blame
the public or the legal profession for calling attention to the failure
of companies to test their products adequately.

Still, even products which have been tested for long periods of
time occasionally run into legal problems. Ortho Pharmaceutical
Company had to pay damages of $5,151,030 as a result of a Georgia
decision in 1986. In this case a woman who had used the spermicide
Ortho-Gyno while she was unaware of being pregnant, alleged that
this caused her baby's birth defects.[8] Though according to Djerassis,
it is highly unlikely that the Ortho spermicide caused the defects,
users of this contraceptive are now warned to avoid using spermicides
if a pregnancy is "suspected." They should also be advised that when
planning a pregnancy, use of spermicides should be avoided for several
days before the most fertile period.[9]

Even the pill has not escaped legal action. As indicated in chapter
4 on oral contraceptives, the pill is not for everyone, and its nature
has changed since first being introduced. Nevertheless, lawsuits are

still brought against the manufacturers. Of the suits focusing on the pill, almost all the cases that have gone to trial have been won by the drug companies, but there have often been out-of-court settlements to avoid the high cost of litigation. Still, in 1982, the Office of Technology Assessment stated that the liability costs in the oral contraception field were higher than that for any other drug product.[10] When is a legal suit justified? Obviously, there is no question that the cases emerging from the Dalkon Shield were warranted, but it is not always clear that cases involving other contraceptives always are. Djerassi is right to emphasize that litigation has been costly, but this cost is usually passed on to the consumer. For example, the cost of a monthly regimen of the pill has increased nearly tenfold in the United States during the past dozen years even though most of the pills on the U.S. market have been "off patent" for many years and available to others. The generic versions of the pill, which finally appeared in 1988, are manufactured by the producers of the proprietary formulations.

Litigation has probably also prevented the introduction of pills with new ingredients from appearing in the United States (although not elsewhere). Three new formulations—desogestrel, norgestimate, and gestodene—were introduced into Europe in the 1980s, but they still have not reached the United States. The leading European manufacturer of the most advanced pill, Desogestrel, has stated that the product has not been introduced into the U.S. market because of potential liability exposure.

Though the long-term monetary gains lie in development of more effective contraceptives, research money invested by the pharmaceutical industry in the United States has declined. Unfortunately, so has the contribution of the federal government. Under President Ronald Reagan, funds for contraceptive research were severely curtailed and they have not yet been given a high priority. Both the National Institutes of Health and the Agency for International Development were prevented from supporting many important areas of contraceptive research that they once encouraged.

This failure to provide adequate funding for contraceptive research has made some social problems worse. For instance, though abortion is a controversial issue in the United States, the government and others have failed to recognize that abortion reflects the current state of contraception. The greater the availability and knowledge of contraceptives, the less likely abortion is to occur. Unfortunately, some of the same groups who are opposed to abortion are also opposed to the use of contraceptives as well as to adequate sex education classes. In the Soviet Union, the country with the highest abortion rate, the quality of birth control is exceedingly poor. In Japan, the country with the third or fourth highest abortion rate, the pill is not approved for contraceptive use. The United States has the highest rate of teenage pregnancy and abortion of any industrialized country and yet those who frustrate sex education efforts make it next to impossible to reach this audience with contraceptive information.

Though there undoubtedly will be improvements in the next few years in existing contraceptive methods with the introduction of another vaginal spermicide tablet, another copper IUD, and other types of cervical caps, there is little chance that any radical new breakthroughs will occur in the United States unless much more money is put into research.

In a sense, however, this state of affairs is not so unusual; Americans traditionally have been very ambivalent about contraceptives. Much of the early contraceptive research, even when it was funded by American groups such as the Rockefeller Foundation or the Population Council, took place outside of the United States because American scientists and companies were unwilling to be involved. This changed in the 1960s and 1970s as not only private foundations but pharmaceutical companies and the federal government entered the field. Much of this money dried up in the 1980s during the Reagan years, and it is just now beginning to be reconsidered. Among the projects that should be funded and are theoretically possible to achieve, five should have priority.

1. One of the most important is a reliable ovulation predictor. Large numbers of couples want to use a natural family planning method, yet all the methods so far available cannot predict when ovulation will occur, though they can indicate that it has occurred. Precisely for this reason family planning methods require a longer period of abstention from sexual intercourse than many people are willing to tolerate. Such prediction is technically feasible, but what needs to be done is to convert this feasibility into an operationally practical method for routine birth control. This would require a considerable investment of time and money, probably by the federal government and foundations since very little benefit would accrue to any pharmaceutical company from such research.

2. More profitable, desirable, and theoretically possible is the development of a once-a-month pill for inducing menstruation. To be valuable for large numbers of women, it would need to be self-administered and not be accompanied by serious side effects. RU 486 is a step in this direction but more work needs to be done.

3. Of great significance is the development of an easily reversible and reliable method of male sterilization. This is a difficult problem for reasons we have already discussed (see chapter 9), but it is a problem that needs to be explored in greater detail. Some effort is being made in this direction but it still remains only theoretically possible. Much needed also is a male contraceptive pill. Since the developer would gain financially, this is a project that could be shared with the pharmaceutical companies.

4. A major breakthrough would be the development of an anti-fertility vaccine. If it was possible to vaccinate teenage males and females so that they would be infertile until a conscious step was taken to achieve fertility, our whole concept of fertility would change and certainly our concerns about teenagers would be different. The search for a vaccine effective for females has been underway for well over a decade but it will take many years of careful, controlled studies with large numbers of female volunteers to determine how long it takes for the effect of the antifertility vaccine to wear off, whether all women are then able to produce normal healthy babies, and whether there are serious side effects. Efforts have also been underway to seek a male vaccine, but progress in this direction has proven much slower.

5. High on the priority list in this age of AIDS is the development of a new spermicide with better antiviral properties. It would not only enable society to win its battle against AIDS, but it would help to cut down the incidence of other sexually transmitted diseases. Again, this is a theoretical possibility that needs considerable money and effort to develop fully, and it could be a joint effort of private and public agencies and companies.

In sum, there have been major breakthroughs in the last thirty years, but there is a need for many more; and, in addition, we need a higher prioritization of research in the area of contraceptives. The effect of all the discoveries, however, has been to lessen the importance of the sexual act as simply one of procreation and to emphasize the pleasurable aspects of sex. The result has been a radical change in attitudes and behaviors, which even the AIDS epidemic has not changed. It is the fear of such changes in behavior that has been the major barrier to contraceptive research in the past and still works to handicap research today, much more so than any threat of legal action or the demand of the government for adequate testing.

NOTES

1. Based on R. A. Hatcher, F. Guest, F. Stewart, G. K. Stewart, J. Trussell, S. C. Bowen, and W. Cates, *Contraceptive Technology: 1988–1989,* 14th rev. ed. (New York: Irvington Publishers, 1988), p. 151.

2. Ibid, p. 157.

3. *Understanding AIDS,* U.S. Department of Health and Human Services, Publication No. (CDC) HHS–88–8404 (Washington D.C.: U.S. Government Printing Office, 1988).

4. I. L. Reiss, and R. L. Leik, "Evaluating Strategies to Avoid AIDS: Number of Partners vs. Use of Condoms," *The Journal of Sex Research* 26 (November 1989): 411–33

5. Carl Djerassi, "Birth Control After 1984," *Science* 169 (1970): 1941.

6. See Carl Djerassi, "The Bitter Pill," *Science* 245 (July 28, 1989): 356–61.

7. Morton Mintz, *At Any Cost: Corporate Greed, Women, and the Dalkon Shield* (New York: Pantheon Books, 1988).

8. *Wells* v. *Ortho Pharmaceutical Co.,* 615 F. Supp. 262 (N.D. GA 1985), aff'd, 788 F. 2d 741 (11th Cir. 1986).

9. "Warning on Spermicides," *Newsweek* (April 13, 1989): 84.

10. *World Population and Fertility Planning Technologies—The Next 20 Years* (Washington, D.C.: Congress of the United States, Office of Technology Assessment, 1982).

Index